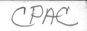

coconut oil for
health and beauty

coconut oil for health and beauty

Uses, Benefits, and Recipes for Weight Loss, Allergies, and Healthy Skin and Hair

Simone McGrath

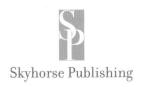

Skyhorse Publishing

Skyhorse Publishing books may be purchased in bulk at special discounts for sales promotion, corporate gifts, fund-raising, or educational purposes. Special editions can also be created to specifications. For details, contact the Special Sales Department, Skyhorse Publishing, 307 West 36th Street, 11th Floor, New York, NY 10018 or info@skyhorsepublishing.com.

Skyhorse® and Skyhorse Publishing® are registered trademarks of Skyhorse Publishing, Inc.®, a Delaware corporation.

www.skyhorsepublishing.com

10 9 8 7 6 5 4 3 2 1

Library of Congress Cataloging-in-Publication Data is available on file.

ISBN: 978-1-62873-752-3

Printed in China

contents

.... contents ....

.... contents ....

.... contents ....

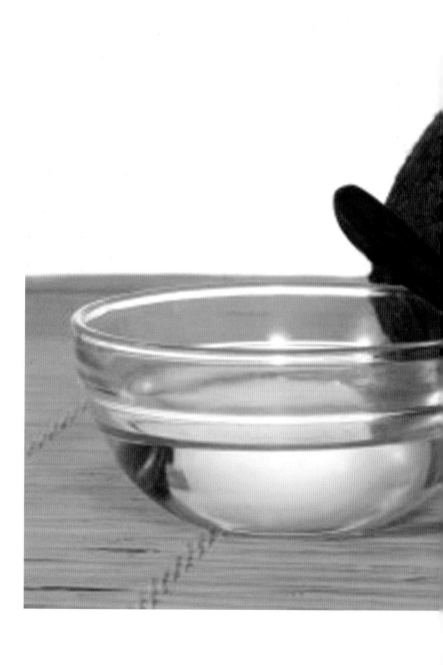

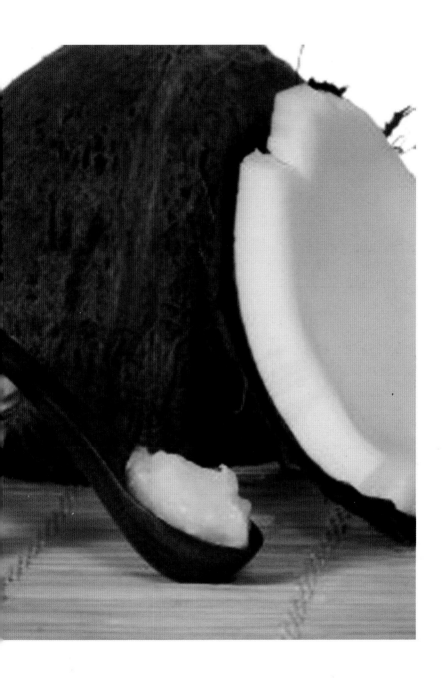

Introduction to Coconut Oil

Lately, coconut oil has received a great deal of attention as a highly versatile wonder-food capable of working as the base of healthy nutrition, natural medication, and beauty products. So is all the hype true?

Many people have reported miraculous health benefits from using this amazing oil, while doctors and scientists are also showing a renewed interest in the possibilities of coconut oil due to its unique chemical composition.

Coconut oil is composed of mainly healthy fats, which are extremely beneficial to our health, particularly to our hearts and our weight. Meals and snacks containing coconut oil, such as coconut smoothies, are popular across the world as help shed some extra pounds. Coconut oil also contains lauric acid, which has powerful immune-strengthening properties, making it capable of curbing the symptoms of the common cold and even fighting diseases caused by serious immune deficiencies. A healthy intake of coconut oil will boost your immunity so you will thrive year-round.

Coconut oil not only makes you feel healthier, but also makes you look better too. Regular applications of coconut oil will make your hair and skin healthier, softer, and brighter than ever. Many people spend huge sums on cleansing ointments, anti-aging creams, and acne treatment, only to be disappointed. Little do they realize that the coconut oil in the next supermarket aisle actually contains greater cleansing, healing, and moisturizing properties than the commercial products in the beauty aisle.

So yes, it is true! This book will explain exactly why coconut oil is nature's most versatile gift, and we will show you how to use it in cooking, and beauty therapy and as a medicinal treatment.

The Tree of Life

Coconut oil, of course, comes from a coconut—arguably the most versatile, nutritious, and therapeutic natural food on the planet! The coconut is not actually a nut. It is botanically classified as a drupe, which is a fruit with a breakable fault-line where it splits easily. Coconuts are the fruit of the coconut palm, which is native to Malaysia, Polynesia, and southern Asia. Now it is also found in tropical climates throughout the world, particularly the Philippines, Vanuatu, and India, as well as some parts of South America and Australia. This is to the popularity of the coconut as trading currency and to the ability of the husk to float across oceans where it propagates on other tropical islands. Now almost one-third of the world's population relies on the coconut for food and trade.

In literature, the coconut was first mentioned in the tales of Sinbad the Sailor recorded in *The Arabian Nights*. Sinbad is briefly shipwrecked on an island, where he discovers a huge crop of coconuts. Once his ship is repaired, he loads it up with coconuts and has a pleasant voyage home, stopping at various islands to trade them along his way. Historically, coconuts were valuable trade commodities in the Indian Ocean's Nicobar Islands well into the twentieth century.

Marco Polo mentioned the *nux indica* ("Indian nut") he discovered in Sumatra during the thirteenth century. Sir Francis Drake called the fruit "nargils." It is believed that Portuguese explorers originated the name *coconut* from their word *coco*, meaning "grinning face" or "monkey face" because the three indentations on top of the coconut resemble a face.

The Sanskrit term for the coconut palm is *kalpa vriksha*, meaning "tree which gives all that is necessary for living," or "The Tree of Life" because the tree and fruit provide material for food, shelter, medicine, and fuel. The coconut provides meat, water, milk, and oil; these can be consumed directly or used as ingredients for meals, medicines, soaps, and cosmetics. Coconut water contains a high level of electrolytes and is hygienic and therapeutic enough to be administered intravenously—during both World War II and the Vietnam War, doctors used coconut water as an intravenous solution when medical supplies ran out. The husk contains a fiber called coir, which was traditionally used as fuel and is now used to make ropes, matting, padding, or upholstery. Some South Pacific islanders even carved the shell into small discs to use as coins. The tree itself can be used for fuel or building shelter; however, as it bears fruit thirteen times a year, it is better to keep harvesting all those coconuts! Since the tree continually bears fruit year-round, it is rarely chopped down, so coconuts are an environmentally friendly source of nutrition.

The versatility of the coconut is not the only reason it has remained so popular and valuable for centuries. The coconut is also rich in essential nutrients and has magnificent healing properties. Coconut oil, a natural extract of the coconut, has been dubbed "the healthiest oil on Earth." What other substance can soothe eczema, improve dental hygiene, decrease the risk of heart disease, cure dandruff, increase immunity, and improve digestion? Coconut oil is indeed an amazing product of the "Tree of Life."

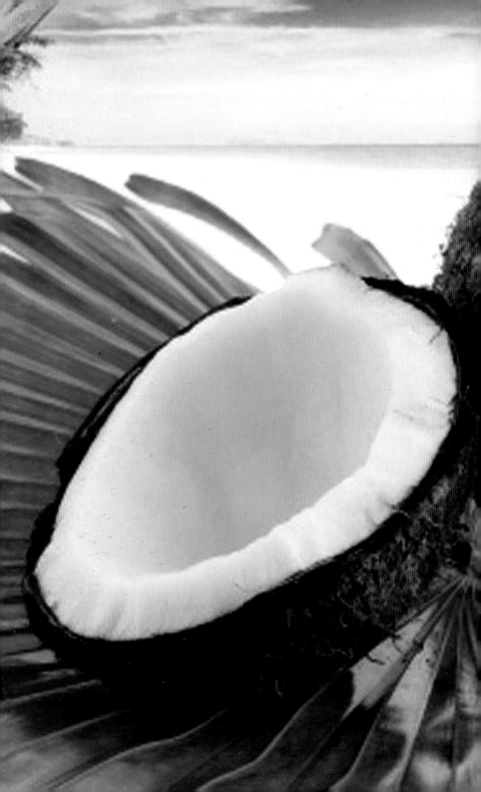

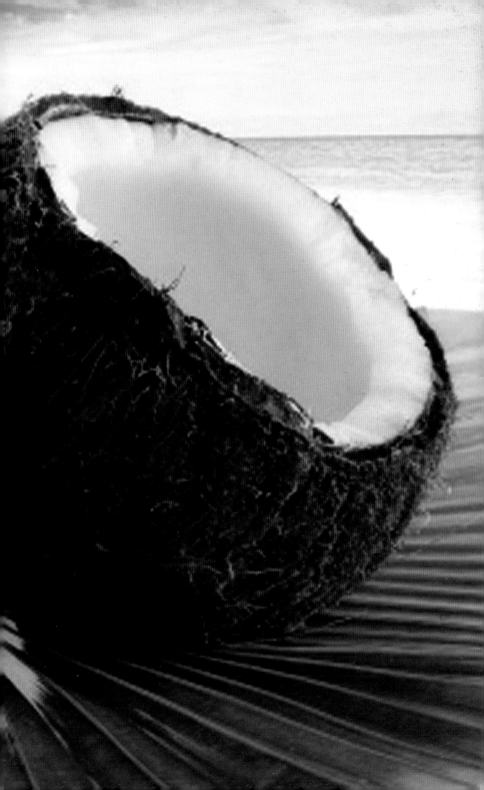

How to Break a Coconut

There is so much goodness hidden inside a coconut—but it is not that easy to release this goodness from within the hard outer shell! When opening a coconut for the first time, you risk injuring yourself or losing some of the nutritious content in the process.

Imagine the coconut is a world globe. The coconut has a soft "eye" at the North Pole and a natural breaking line along the Equator.

First, locate the eye at the top of the coconut. This eye is much softer than the rest of the coconut shell, so you can slide a metal skewer or a knife through to make a hole. Be careful not to lose your grip on the coconut while sliding the sharp implement through the shell. If your hand slips, you risk cutting yourself.

Once you have penetrated the shell, drain the coconut water into a jug. Now work out where the Equator would run around your coconut. Tap gently around it with a hammer, or thump the coconut against a wall until the coconut splits open. If your coconut is particularly stubborn, place it into a plastic bag and hit it directly with a hammer. When the coconut finally comes apart, it will all be neatly contained in the plastic bag.

Modern Coconut Harvesting

Traditional tropical island life was fairly simple and uncomplicated: the basic method of collecting coconuts by climbing or shaking a tree and then breaking them to reach the copra (coconut meat) would be enough to provide the local village with all the coconut meat, milk, and oil they required. The meat would be scooped out by hand and ground into a paste, creating a thick version of coconut milk. However, when Pacific Islanders recognized the valuable international interest in the coconut, they realized they needed to modernize their methods of extracting the precious coconut oil from copra to meet demand.

The most important and innovative advance in coconut harvesting was the dehusking machine, which was first created in the nineteenth century. The dehusking machine neatly removes the husk from around the meat of the coconut, eliminating the arduous task of cracking open the husk and scooping out the hard meat with a knife or sharp stick. It extracts the copra faster and more efficiently than a person can manually—a modern dehusking machine can dehusk three-hundred coconuts in an hour with minimal wastage of copra.

Interestingly, modern coconut farmers still practice the traditional method of grinding the copra. Most coconut oil producers will ferment the ground white pulp in bulk tanks for roughly seventy-two hours. Sitting undisturbed, the thick milk separates into water and oil, doing almost all the work independently.

What Is Virgin Coconut Oil?

You'll see different labels on the supermarket shelves—coconut oil, virgin coconut oil, and extra-virgin coconut oil. So what's the difference?

Basic (or "refined") coconut oil is made from dried copra. Most coconuts are sourced from remote villages far away from copra mills where the copra is processed into oil. It is a long journey to the copra mill, so villagers will smoke the copra to keep it longer. Then, after a few months, they deliver a large supply to the mill. The copra is generally smoke-dried but can also be sun-dried or kiln-dried. Smoke-dried copra looks dirty and has a rancid taste, so it must be bleached and cleaned with chemicals.

Virgin coconut oil is made from fresh copra. While villagers will toil for months to smoke enough copra to take to the mill, they will use a few fresh coconuts to whip up some virgin coconut oil for their own use. The virgin coconut oil is completely pure—it requires only minimal heating and no refining. It is higher quality and more expensive than standard coconut oil because of course it is more time-consuming to make large quantities of oil from fresh coconuts.

Some unscrupulous companies will label their bottles "virgin" or even "extra virgin" if the product is derived from dried copra. As there is no industry standard definition for virgin coconut oil, these companies can get away with falsely labeling their products. The best way to distinguish virgin coconut oil from standard coconut oil is to smell it. The purest, cleanest coconut oil still has the aroma of fresh coconut.

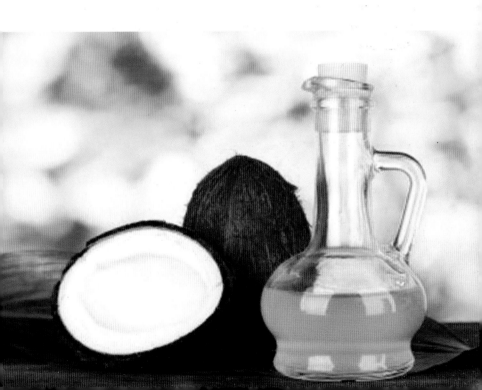

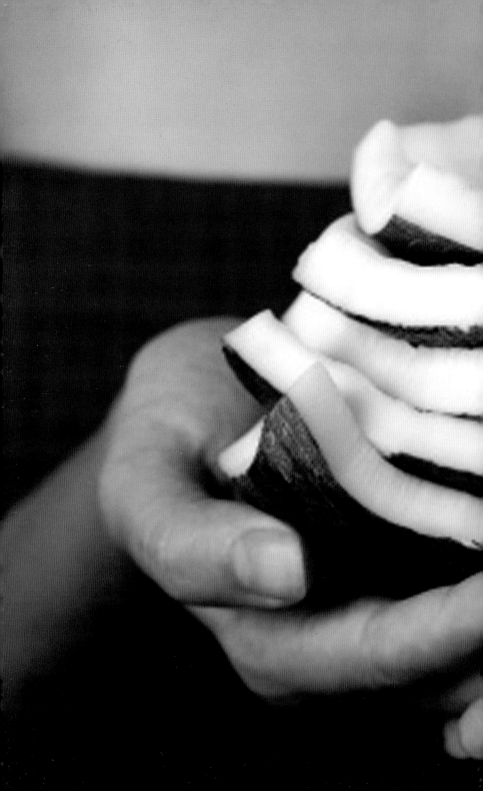

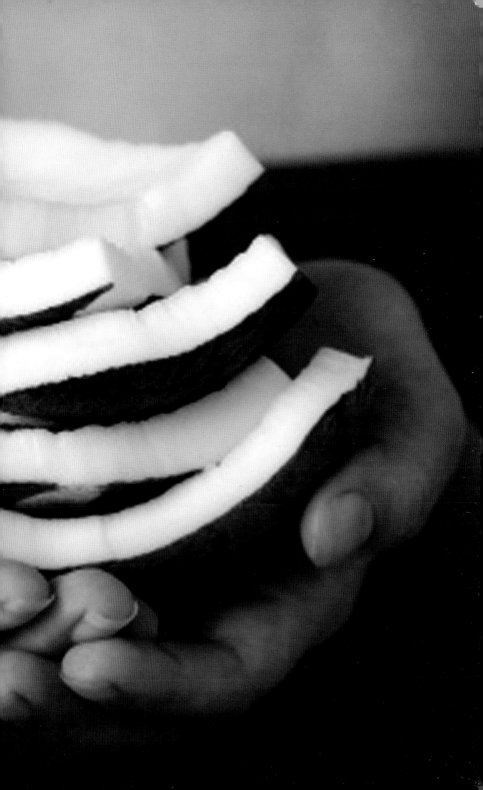

Dietary Benefits of Coconut Oil

The website of the Coconut Research Center (www.coconut-researchcenter.org) includes countless testimonials from people who have dramatically improved their health with a daily spoonful of coconut oil. Seventy-six-year-old Diana took regular doses of coconut oil when she was diagnosed with diabetes, and her blood sugar levels improved dramatically; Charlie B. attributes coconut oil to lowering his high blood pressure; and Giovanna wrote that her husband was due to have surgery to control debilitating ulcerative colitis, but his health improved dramatically when a friend recommended coconut oil.

You don't need to swallow coconut oil to benefit from its healing powers: a young mother named Nellita wrote in to say she has successfully cured her daughter's eczema by applying coconut oil on the skin. One man wrote that his teeth and gums have improved since he began "oil pulling." Other coconut oil fans describe improvements to their hair, their skin, even their sex lives!

Is it all true? Is there any scientific basis to these claims that coconut oil can cure so many ailments?

The rejuvenating properties of coconut oil are due to a unique blend of saturated fatty acids. Medical studies show that a daily intake of coconut oil can help our bodies mount resistance to both viruses and bacteria, thereby helping us withstand illness and disease. Coconut oil also helps fight off yeast, fungus, and Candida overgrowth in the body and has a positive effect on our hormones, helping us naturally balance our thyroid levels and increasing our metabolism and energy levels. As coconuts help the body use insulin more efficiently, coconut oil also helps maintain healthy blood sugar levels. It also stimulates digestion and absorbs fat-soluble vitamins, so you absorb more nutrients from your daily diet.

You don't need to be ill to investigate the health properties of coconut oil. It can cleanse your hair and skin, adding a healthy glow that will enhance your appearance and well-being.

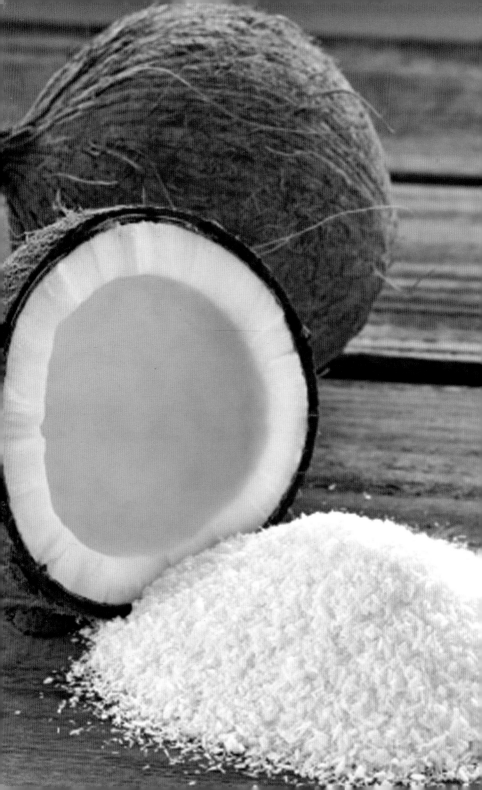

The Fatty Acids in Coconut Oil

Coconut oil contains a blend of three fatty acids—lauric acid, capric acid, and caprylic acid. Fatty acids are an essential source of fuel for the body and the brain. Individually, each of these fatty acids has important healing powers. Combined, they are even more effective!

Capric acid, also known as decanoic acid, is the central reason for the health-giving properties of coconut oil. The word *capric* comes from the Latin word for goat, as capric acid is found in goat's milk. It is also found in cow's milk, although only coconut oil and palm oil contain capric acid in substantial quantities.

Capric acid combines with lauric acid and caprylic acid to trigger an increase in high-density lipoprotein (HDL) or "good" cholesterol. The "good" cholesterol lowers the risk of artherosclerosis, or thickening of the artery wall, a common and potentially fatal condition with no symptoms.

Capric acid has other beneficial properties. Once ingested, it converts into monocaprin, a substance with the ability to fight viruses, bacteria, and yeast infections such as Candida albicans. Monocaprin is also believed to help you release energy more efficiently, so you can remain active longer. It can be argued that in the longterm, capric acid can trigger weight loss and improve fitness.

Caprylic acid, is also found naturally in goat's milk and cow's milk as well as in coconut oil. Caprylic acid is believed to be effective in combating yeast infections and fighting bacteria such as staphylococcus and streptococcus. It is also believed to work as an antifungal agent by interfering with the cell walls of fungal infections such as Candida albicans. Caprylic acid will balance stomach acidity, and this in turn boosts the immune system, so you fight infection more effectively.

Lauric acid is a saturated fatty acid suitable for the production of soaps and cosmetics. Once ingested, it converts into mono-laurin, a substance with strong antibacterial properties found only in human breastmilk and coconut oil. Monolaurin works to eliminate lipid-coated viruses such as herpes and influenza.

About two-thirds of the fatty acids in coconut oil are medium-chain fatty acids (MCFAs), making coconut oil the world's richest source of MCFAs. Vegetable oils and seed oils contain long-chain fatty acids (LCFAs), which are difficult to digest, so they are stored as cholesterol or fat. MCFAs are smaller than LCFAs, so they penetrate cell walls more easily, and unlike LCFAs, they convert into energy rather than fat.

Coconut oil can boost your metabolism both by providing more energy and by stimulating your thyroid gland. With a more efficient metabolism, you will heal faster and bounce back from illness better.

Saturated Fat and "Good" Cholesterol

You might be wondering why we are talking about coconut oil as healthy, when clearly *fatty acids* is another term for "saturated fat." Saturated fat is *unhealthy*, isn't it?

Actually, naturally occurring saturated fat is extremely healthy for you. Artificially created saturated fat—also known as trans fat—is not. Food distributors add extra hydrogen atoms to unsaturated products such as vegetable oil or seed oil in a process called hydrogenation so the products will last longer.

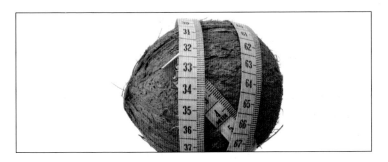

Hydrogenation transforms the healthy and natural unsaturated fat into unhealthy unnatural saturated fat and ruins the reputation of natural saturated fats such as coconut oil.

For decades (since the introduction of hydrogenation and trans fats), saturated fat has been blamed for health conditions such as cardiovascular disease. But Pacific Islanders, who incorporate coconut oil into almost all their meals, have an extremely low incidence of cardiovascular disease and other health issues related to saturated fat. This is partly due to the combined presence of capric, lauric, and caprylic acids, which boost the production of lipoprotein, the "good" cholesterol that improves the health of your heart.

So the myth that coconut oil is bad for you is actually an intentional clouding over of the true message that artificially created saturated fat is unhealthy for you. Coconut oil, as a natural product, containing natural substances rarely found in other foods, is extremely beneficial for your overall health and well-being.

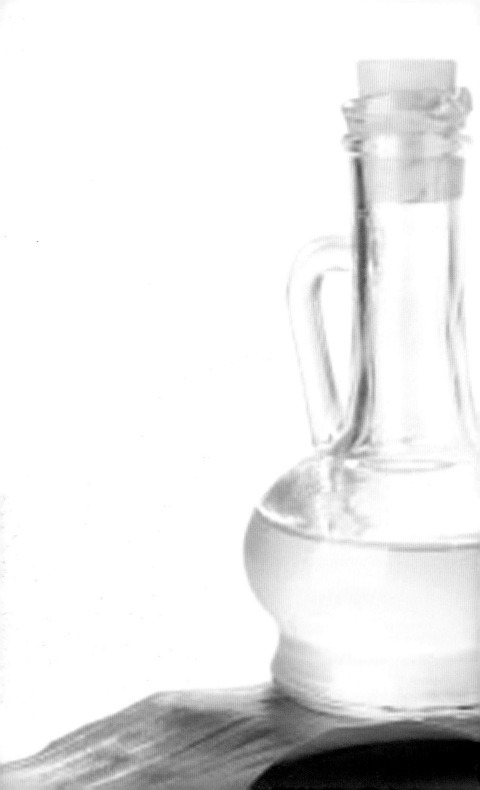

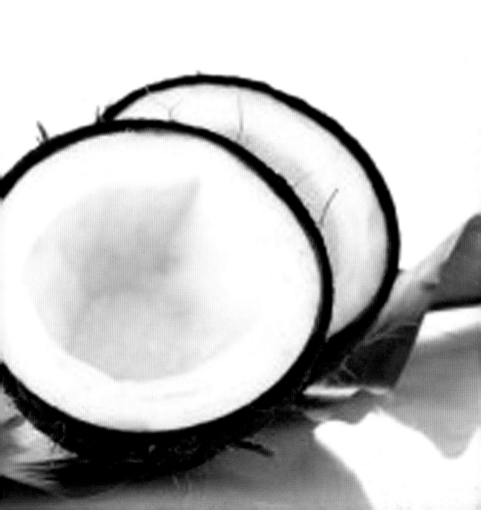

How to Make Coconut Oil at Home

Makes approximately 6.5 oz (200 ml) of oil
You will need:

- 3 coconuts
- A sharp cleaver
- Metal spoon/paring knife
- Food processor (or grater)
- Sheet of cheesecloth
- Bowl
- Glass jar with lid

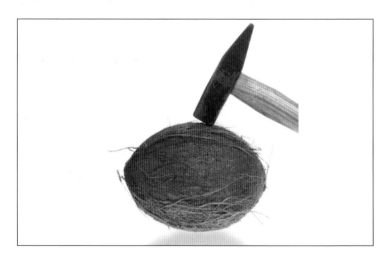

First, split your coconuts with the cleaver, very carefully. Have a bowl handy, so as the coconut cracks open, you can save the coconut water that is stored in the center of the coconut. Coconut water is a cloudy, watery fluid, rich in electrolytes, so it is healthy to drink.

Once you have opened the coconut, you will see the shell is lined with a thick white layer. This is the coconut "meat." Use a metal spoon to scrape all the meat from the shell. If you need some extra help, try using a paring knife. When you have removed all the meat from the shell, slice it into small pieces. Put these pieces into the food processor and blend at medium seed until the meat is pulpy.

Cover a bowl with cheesecloth and spoon a portion of the coconut mixture onto the cheesecloth. Then wrap the cloth around the coconut and squeeze the bundle over the bowl. You will see coconut milk drain through the cloth into the bowl. Keep squeezing until you have removed all the fluid from the pulp, then put the pulp aside and spoon another batch of coconut mixture into the cheesecloth. Repeat until you have squeezed all the fluid from the mixture.

Now pour the fluid into a glass jar and secure the lid. Leave it to ferment for forty-eight hours.

Set the jar aside until you see a thick layer of curd has appeared at the top of the jar. Once the curd has risen, place the jar in the fridge so the curd can harden.

Once the curd has hardened, you can remove it with a spoon, and the remaining thick liquid in the jar is your coconut oil.

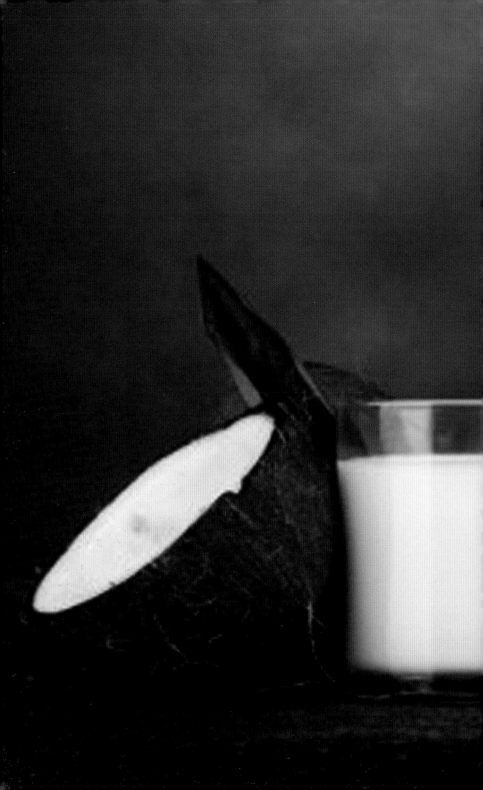

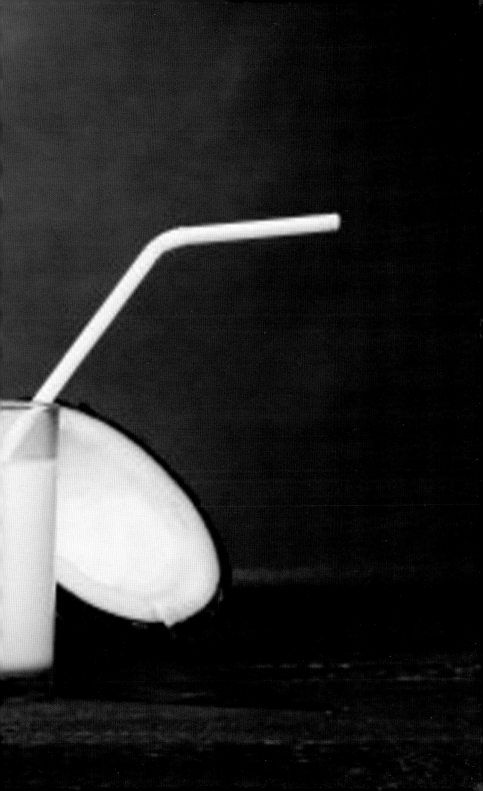

How to Make Your Own Fresh Coconut Milk or Cream

While coconut milk is always available in the supermarket, nothing beats the nutritious and delicious value of your own freshly made coconut milk.

Ingredients:

A fresh coconut (preferably an organic one) or 1 cup dried shredded coconut

A good quality grater (or food processor with grater attachment)

A cheesecloth, fine mesh strainer, or nut milk bag (you can easily find these in a health food shop)

Hot water (preferably purified)

A good-quality blender

If using fresh coconut, grate all the flesh. Be sure to remove the brown outer skin.

If using shredded coconut, put equal parts of coconut and purified water in a bowl and let it soak and rehydrate.

Place 1 cup of your grated/hydrated coconut in a blender with 2 cups of warm water and blend until smooth. For a creamier texture, use less water.

Pour through a fine mesh strainer, cheesecloth, or nut milk bag.

Repeat the process with the remaining coconut in the strainer. Do not repeat too many times, as the milk will be weaker each time. Leftover coconut meal can be baked in to cookies.

Enjoy this fresh coconut milk or coconut cream in your smoothies, curries, healthy desserts, or anywhere a recipe calls for coconut milk or coconut cream.

Storing Coconut Milk and Coconut Cream

As fresh coconut milk/cream has a short shelf life, you should use it immediately or freeze in BPA-free food containers, ice cube trays, or baby-food storage containers. Ice cube trays give you the correct portions and temperature for fresh smoothies!

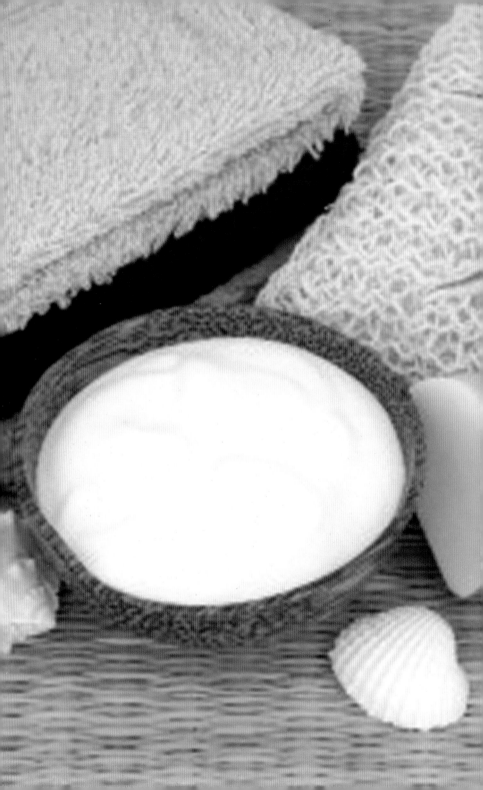

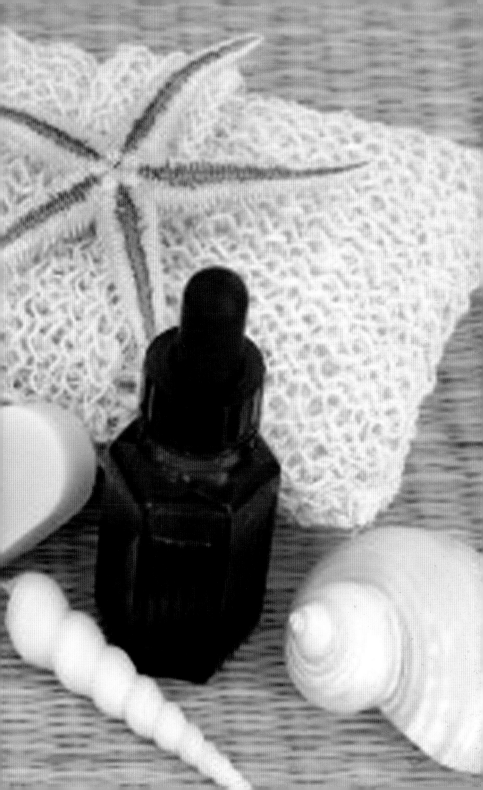

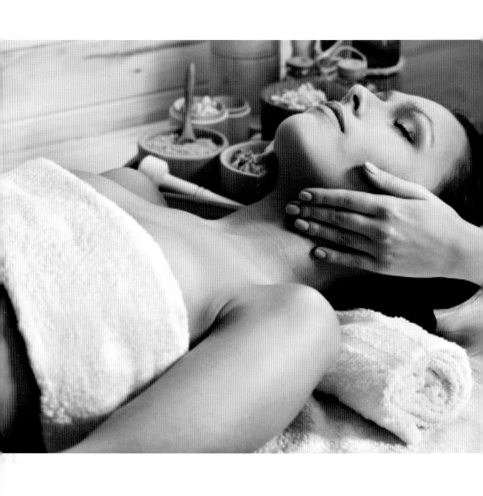

Coconut Oil as Beauty Therapy

Coconut oil is a unique and effective all-in-one beauty tool, ideal for your skin, your hair, and even your teeth! The beauty industry is well aware of the cleansing and moisturizing properties of this versatile substance, so it is a regular ingredient in expensive lotions, soaps, and shampoos. However, commercial beauty products also include chemicals acting as preservatives and artificial fragrance—so why spend enormous amounts when you can achieve a better result for the small cost of coconut oil?

We will show you how coconut oil can replace all those little jars and bottles in your bathroom cabinet to soothe, nourish, and cleanse your whole family.

Skin Care with Coconut Oil

Pure virgin coconut oil is the ideal cleanser and moisturizer for your skin. Unlike commercial cleansers and moisturizers, it will not strip your skin of its natural layer of protection. As coconut oil contains a high level of fats, it is also an excellent emollient, smoothing your skin to remove fine lines and soothing itching and irritation. It can moisturize your skin so it is supple and glowing, and the nutrients in coconut oil will rejuvenate and nourish new cells while removing dead skin cells.

Coconut oil is a highly effective treatment for skin conditions such as acne, dermatitis, eczema, and psoriasis. Once coconut oil has absorbed into the skin, it disrupts the natural environment for microbes that trigger such skin conditions. Coconut oil also has healing powers due to its antiseptic properties, so it speeds healing of acne, rashes, and even minor cuts and wounds.

Skin Care Recipes

Coconut Bath Melts

This makes a great personal gift or just your own private bath-time indulgence.

Equipment:

    Double boiler saucepan
    Jug

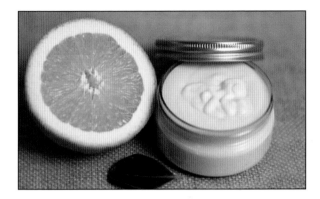

Glass bowl

Decorative molds—a decorative ice-cube tray is ideal. If you use a normal ice cube tray, you can consider cutting each mold into two.

Glass storage jar

Ingredients:

2 teaspoons of cocoa butter

2 teaspoons of coconut oil

2 tablespoons of sweet almond oil

1 teaspoon of jojoba oil

Approximately 6 drops of essential oil of your choice

This amount should fill one ice cube tray or equivalent

Heat water in the lower section of the double boiler, then melt cocoa butter and coconut oil and stir together in the top section. Stir gently until they are completely combined. Add the liquid oils. Pour into the jug. Add essential oils to provide the desired scent. Fill each mold with the melted and scented oil, then place the tray in the fridge for a few hours until they are completely solid.

Store the bath melts in a glass jar in a cool cupboard. When you're ready for a soothing and refreshing bath, drop one or two bath melts into the running water.

Whipped Coconut Oil Body Butter

Only a small amount of this luxurious all-over moisturizer will leave your skin glowing and replenished, soft, and smooth.

Equipment:

Electric hand mixer or stand mixer
Mixing bowl
Glass jar with sealed lid

Ingredients:

1 cup solid coconut oil
1 teaspoon Vitamin E oil
Approximately 6 drops of essential oils of your choice

Place coconut oil and Vitamin E oil into the mixing bowl. Mix on high speed for about ten minutes, until light and fluffy. Fold in the essential oils. Spoon the body butter into a glass jar and secure the lid.

Store your body butter in a cool place and slather over your skin as required.

Avocado and Coconut Oil Hydrating Face Mask

This face mask will rejuvenate your skin, leaving you feeling fresh and invigorated. The antioxidant properties of honey will enhance coconut oil's natural healing properties. This recipe is for one instant face mask.

Equipment:
  1 bowl
  1 fork
  Electric mixer

Ingredients:
  2 tablespoons virgin coconut oil
  1 tablespoon honey
  ½ avocado
  2 thin slices cucumber (optional)

Mash the avocado with a fork until it is a fairly smooth paste. Add coconut oil and honey, and blend with mixer on a low setting until combined.

Spread the mask over your face and neck, avoiding the eyes. Place cucumber slices over your eyes to rejuvenate the delicate skin. Keep the mask on for fifteen to twenty minutes then wash off thoroughly with warm water.

Honey and Coconut Oil Healing Mask

This mask combines the healing properties of coconut oil and honey with the antioxidant properties and smooth texture of Greek yogurt, making it ideal for anyone suffering from acne or dermatitis. It must be applied within a few hours of making it to ensure the ingredients remain fresh and potent.

Equipment:
  Bowl
  Hand-held mixer

Ingredients:
  1 tablespoon honey

1 tablespoon Greek yogurt
1 tablespoon virgin coconut oil
1 teaspoon arrowroot
5 drops of lemon juice *or* 3 drops tea tree oil

Place all ingredients in bowl and mix gently until well combined. If you don't plan to use the mask straight away, refrigerate it in a covered container.

To apply, smooth it over the T-zone, working down from the forehead. Then make a second application over the entire face and neck. Avoid the area around the eyes. Leave on for approximately fifteen minutes then wash off thoroughly with warm water.

Coconut Peppermint Body Scrub

This invigorating scrub will exfoliate your skin, leaving you feeling fresh and glowing. It is suitable for use up to three times a week. If you prefer, you can choose another essential oil other than peppermint.

Equipment:
Bowl
Wooden spoon
Measuring spoon
Container with lid

Ingredients:
2 tablespoons virgin coconut oil
Pinch of sea salt
2 tablespoons brown sugar

Approximately 1 tablespoon orange juice

Approximately 6 drops peppermint

Mix the dry ingredients then add sufficient orange juice to attain the desired texture. Store in jar and keep in a cool place.

To apply, scoop the body scrub into your hand and rub into your body using a circular motion. Concentrate on any particular areas of dry skin. Then wash off the scrub in the shower.

Coconut Oil Antiperspirant Deodorant

While you can choose your own fragrance for this homemade deodorant, you must include grapefruit oil and tea tree oil as they are essential to making the deodorant effective.

Bacteria and microbes thrive in a damp and dark environment, and they are the cause of the unpleasant smell of body odor. Grapefruit neutralizes bacteria and tea tree oil, like coconut oil, eliminates microbes, effectively destroying their ability to create that unpleasant smell. The combination of arrowroot powder and cornstarch helps the deodorant work as an antiperspirant.

Equipment:

Bowl

Fork

Empty roll-on deodorant container

Ingredients:

⅓ cup coconut oil

¼ cup baking soda

¼ cup arrowroot powder

¼ cup cornstarch

1 teaspoon grapefruit juice

3 drops of tea tree oil 5drops of grapefruit oil

A combination of three other essential oils of your choice

Mix the dry ingredients in a bowl, then add coconut oil. Use a fork to combine the coconut oil with the other ingredients. Add essential oils, then add juice slowly until you reach your desired consistency. Pour into roll-on deodorant container. Keep in a cool place.

Coconut and Almond Eye Balm

This soothing and refreshing balm is gentle enough to use on the delicate skin around the eyes. The addition of soybean oil will help eradicate puffiness and dark shadows under the eyes.

Equipment:

Bowl

Metal spoon

Small container with sealed lid

Ingredients:

2 tablespoons coconut oil

1 tablespoon almond oil

1 tablespoon soy bean oil

Blend the three oils gently in a bowl until combined with a consistent texture. Store in a cool place.

To use, apply a small amount of the balm with your finger tip, stroking gently under the eye, and then closing your eye to stroke across the upper lid. You can keep the balm on for better results;

alternately, you can remove it gently using a cotton ball dipped in warm water.

Coconut Oil Pre-Shaving Lotion

Pure virgin coconut oil on its own makes a great lotion to protect your skin from the nicks and irritation of shaving. Stroke softened coconut oil over the area you wish to shave and you will see that the razor glides more easily, leaving your skin soft and silkysmooth. It also prevents ingrown hairs and helps heal skin faster.

Sesame and Coconut (Mild) Sunscreen

When you just want the added protection of a mild SP4 sunscreen while you're out and about, coconut oil is the all-natural solution. While SP4 is a relatively low sun-protection rating, coconut oil has the added bonus of the vitamins and nutrients you need to replenish your skin after exposure to the sun's free radicals. Sesame oil has similar properties, so the two combined make an excellent light natural sunscreen.

Combine 1 cup of coconut oil with 1 cup of sesame oil. Store in a bottle with a tight lid and keep in a cool place.

Coconut Zinc Wax Diaper Rash Cream

This recipe relies on zinc oxide powder as the active ingredient. Zinc oxide has powerful antibacterial and antioxidant properties, removing the irritants that inflame the rash. Like coconut oil, it also contains nutrients that are absorbed into the skin to stimulate healing. The texture of coconut oil ensures that the cream glides smoothly over the skin, so the baby feels better from the start. The beeswax binds the other ingredients together and creates a protective waterproof layer while the baby's skin heals naturally.

Unlike other moisturizing agents, coconut oil keeps the pores open instead of blocking them. So this cream is suitable for any kind of rash and can be used repeatedly to soothe and stimulate healing.

Ingredients:

¼ cup beeswax

1¼ cups virgin coconut oil

1½ teaspoons zinc oxide powder

1 teaspoon arrowroot

Melt beeswax and coconut oil over low heat in the top portion of a double boiler. Pour into a bowl and add dry ingredients. Combine ingredients using an electric mixer. If necessary, add a little more of the coconut oil/beeswax combination or more dry ingredients to achieve the right consistency.

Store in a jar with an airtight lid. Apply small amounts to afflicted area.

Coconut Oil and Dental Care

Coconut oil with its antibacterial properties is ideal for oral hygiene and tooth-whitening. Coconut oil inhibits the growth of bacteria commonly found in the mouth, particularly Streptococcus mutans, the bacteria most responsible for tooth decay.

The simplest way to incorporate coconut oil in your oral hygiene routine is by oil pulling. If you're really keen, you can make your own toothpaste!

Oil Pulling

You wouldn't know from the name, but oil pulling is actually the ancient Indian method of cleansing the mouth and teeth with virgin

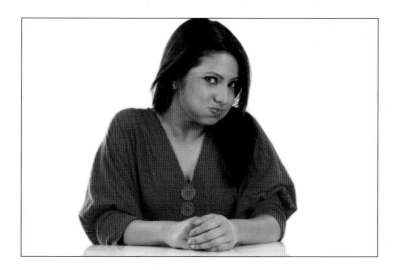

oil. Oil pulling dates back thousands of years as part of Ayurvedic (Sanskrit for "life-knowledge") medicinal practice. It is believed to cleanse your gums and remove toxins and harmful bacteria from your mouth, lowering the risk of tooth decay and disease.

When you swirl the oil in your mouth, all the harmful bacteria and parasites in your mouth bond with the oil, so you can eliminate them once you spit. Coconut oil is ideal for oil pulling, as it contains anti-inflammatory and antimicrobial properties, so it can destroy the hostile bacteria while retaining the probiotics in your mouth.

You will need:

- 1 tablespoon (10 mls) coconut oil
- Disposable container

Swirl the coconut oil around your mouth for five to fifteen minutes. Make sure the oil coats the front and back of your teeth and gums, but keep it away from your throat. **Do not gargle the oil**. The parasites caught in the oil could trigger an infection in your throat.

Once you have thoroughly rinsed your mouth and teeth with coconut oil, spit the oil into a disposable cup and throw the cup away. **Do not spit the coconut oil into the sink or the toilet.** Oils should never enter the plumbing system as they will contaminate water. Coconut oil will also harden and may cause blockage in the drain.

Coconut Bentonite Toothpaste

This recipe combines a range of highly effective natural ingredients to create a pleasant-tasting and refreshing paste that will clean your teeth at least as thoroughly, if not more, than commercial toothpaste!

Besides coconut oil, this paste includes stevia and bentonite clay. Stevia, also known as sweetleaf, is a plant found in both North and South America, renowned for its sweet-tasting leaves. The sweetness of stevia has a faster onset and is longer-lasting than cane sugar, but most importantly it has minimal impact on blood glucose levels, making it an ideal natural alternative to sugar. Therefore, it works as a natural flavoring agent to overcome the taste of baking soda, which helps clean and whiten the teeth.

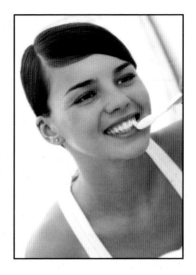

Bentonite clay is derived from volcanic ash and is rich in electrolytes. Its texture enables it to absorb and remove toxins and chemicals. As a toothpaste additive, it can even remove scraps of food from teeth, such as meat. The addition of bentonite clay also makes the texture of homemade toothpaste similar to commercial pastes.

Ingredients:

¼ cup melted coconut oil
2 tablespoons bentonite clay
2 tablespoons baking powder
½ teaspoon Stevia
Peppermint oil to taste

In a mixer, blend all ingredients until well combined. If necessary, adjust the level of coconut oil or dry ingredients until you achieve your desired texture. Adjust the amount of stevia and peppermint oil to achieve your desired taste.

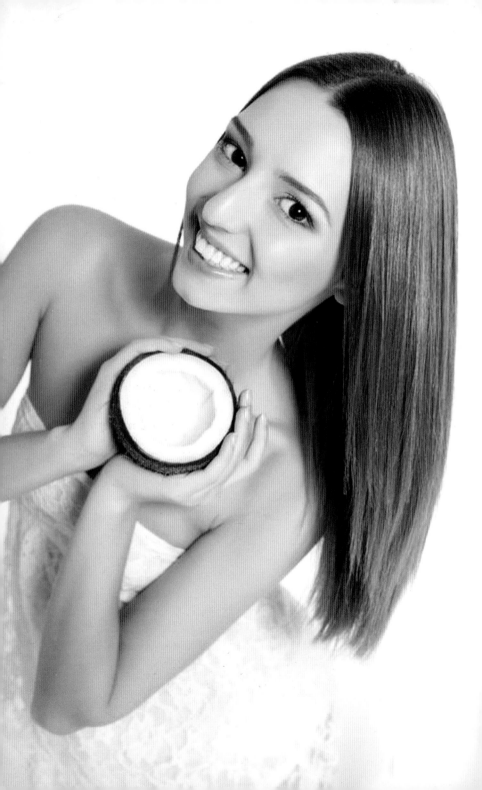

Hair Care with Coconut Oil

Coconut oil will cleanse and strengthen your hair, giving it a natural shine and beautiful condition.

You can apply coconut oil to your hair daily. Massage gently into the scalp, then stroke the oil over your hair. Wash the oil out after thirty minutes. This treatment will keep your scalp healthy and will leave you with strong, lustrous hair. This treatment is particularly recommended for anyone suffering from dandruff or if you have frizzy or brittle hair.

If your hair is extremely damaged and fragile, you can swallow a tablespoon of coconut oil every day, as this will provide you with the nutrients you need to regain your hair's natural strength.

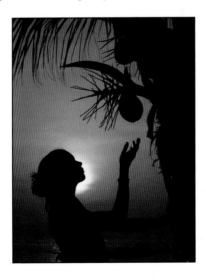

Coconut Oil Hair Care Recipes

For best results, always use virgin coconut oil. All these recipes make enough for one application. For long hair, increase coconut oil by one tablespoon and adjust other ingredients to attain the correct consistency.

Coconut Beer Shampoo

While coconut milk is a very popular shampoo ingredient, coconut oil is usually found in conditioners. However, this shampoo recipe combines coconut oil and beer to give your hair some extra shine and bounce!

Ingredients:

1/4 cup water
1/4 cup liquid Castile soap
1/2 teaspoon melted coconut oil
1 cup beer

Blend water, soap, and oil until well combined. Place beer in a saucepan and bring to the boil over medium heat. Reduce until only 1/4 cup remains. Fold beer into soap mixture until well combined.

Store in a screw-top bottle and keep in a cool place. Use a small amount on hair when showering, and rinse thoroughly.

Deep Conditioning Mask for Normal Hair

Ingredients:

2 tablespoons Manuka honey
2 tablespoons coconut oil
1/4 cup coconut milk
Aromatic essential oils (optional)

Blend coconut oil and honey until well combined. Then fold the coconut milk into the mixture. Apply conditioner to dry hair until all the hair is covered. For best results, wear a shower cap over your hair. Keep the conditioning mask on for thirty to forty-five minutes, then rinse off thoroughly in the shower.

Replenishing Conditioner Treatment for Dry Hair

Ingredients:

1 banana
1 avocado
3 tablespoons coconut oil
2 tablespoons mayonnaise

Mash the banana and avocado thoroughly until smooth and well combined. Stir in the coconut oil and mayonnaise.

Apply treatment to dry hair, ensuring all strands are covered. Keep treatment on for thirty to forty-five minutes. For best results, wear a shower cap. Rinse treatment thoroughly in the shower. Shampooing your hair after the treatment is optional.

Lavender Scalp Cream

If you suffer severely from eczema or dandruff, this scalp cream will remove the dead skin while soothing and healing irritated areas. This recipe also works well as a rejuvenating mask for dry hair.

Ingredients:

>   3 tablespoons coconut oil
>   1 tablespoon olive oil
>   3 drops lavender essential oil (for dry hair mask, replace
> lavender with peppermint)

Melt coconut oil in a double boiler over low heat, and then add olive oil. Once well combined, pour into bowl and add lavender.

Apply to dry hair, ensuring all hair is thoroughly covered. For best results, cover your hair with a shower cap. Keep the treatment on for a minimum of twenty-five minutes. If the scalp is severely inflamed, you can wear the mask all night.

Rinse hair under the shower. Repeat the mask every few days until scalp is healed.

Lemon Pepper Anti-Dandruff Mask

Equipment:

>   Double boiler
>   Muslin straining cloth

Ingredients:

>   2 tablespoons coconut oil
>   ¼ teaspoon black pepper
>   3 drops lemon juice
>   3 drops lavender oil

Heat coconut oil in the top section of a double boiler over low heat until it melts. Remove from heat and add black pepper. Strain the mixture by pouring it through a muslin cloth, then add lemon juice and lavender oil. Stir until well combined. Set aside until the coconut oil is warm but still liquid.

Massage the oil deeply into your scalp. Apply any remaining oil onto your hair by stroking downward. Rub the tips so they are thoroughly covered with the oil. For best results, wear a shower cap over the mask and keep it on for a minimum of thirty minutes, or overnight if possible. Rinse off in cool water under the shower.

Apple Coconut Lice Treatment

Lice are insidious, contagious creatures with strong survival instincts. They travel from person to person through direct contact and can lay hundreds of eggs a day. Within ten days of hatching, they are ready to start their own families. So eliminating lice completely takes two strategies—you need to remove the lice themselves and you must remove all their eggs so you don't have another infestation two weeks later.

Just washing your hair won't get rid of them, as they instinctively close up to protect themselves from water. Their eggs are attached firmly to hairs with a type of natural concrete, so simply combing won't remove the eggs. Their breeding cycle is so rapid that they soon become immune to the toxic commercial treatments available.

However, lice do have their vulnerabilities. They breathe through their bodies, so the best way of removing the lice naturally is by applying a hair mask that suffocates the lice. The acetic acid in vinegar will dissolve the concrete substance attaching the eggs to hair.

It is very important to continue the treatment for at least two weeks, even if you use commercial products, as you will face a reinfestation after ten days if you miss a single louse egg. Commercial products can become very irritating to the scalp and damaging to the hair, so coconut oil and apple cider vinegar are ideal natural alternatives, as they will cleanse and nourish the hair.

Ingredients:

20 oz (600 ml) apple cider vinegar
14 oz (425 ml) melted coconut oil, cooled

Equipment:

Metal fine-tooth comb
Cup of boiling water
Cloth for wiping comb

Rinse hair with vinegar and comb for at least twenty minutes, dipping the comb into the boiling water if you encounter a louse. Wipe the comb on the cloth to clear it of any eggs. For best results, comb your child's hair in front of the television so they are distracted from what you are doing.

Allow the vinegar to dry on the hair, and then apply the cooled coconut oil thickly to the scalp and hair, ensuring all hair is covered thoroughly. For best results, ask your child to wear a shower cap as this will contribute to the elimination process. Keep the mask on for at least three hours (not overnight, as the process will disturb your child's sleep).

Rinse coconut oil thoroughly from hair, then repeat the vinegar treatment, combing the hair with apple cider vinegar to remove lice and eggs.

Repeat the complete treatment three days later and another three days after that. If you are no longer seeing lice, then stop the coconut oil treatment and continue with the vinegar treatment every few days for another two weeks. If you see any small lice, repeat the coconut treatment at least once more.

Tea Tree and Coconut Cradle Cap Treatment

Ingredients:

>   2 tablespoons melted coconut oil
>   2 drops tea tree oil
>   ½ teaspoon turmeric powder
>   1 drop lavender oil

Combine all ingredients and apply a small amount gently to a small section of skin. Check that the combination does not cause extra irritation. If this occurs, add more coconut oil to reduce the amount of essential oils. Use a small amount daily to cover the baby's scalp and rinse off in his or her daily bath.

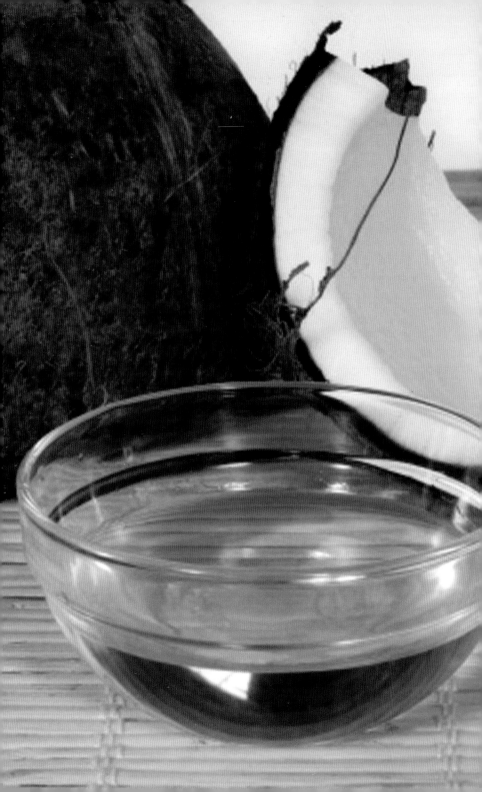

The Therapeutic Powers of Coconut Oil

Coconut oil has been proven to have fantastic healing properties for numerous conditions ranging from Crohn's disease to pneumonia. It also works as a natural preventative medication, shielding your body from viruses and bacteria that would trigger disease, and it can also help reverse or control degenerative conditions such as Alzheimer's disease.

The healthy fat content of coconut oil is one of the reasons it is believed to prevent these conditions. The food industry has been promoting low-fat diets to counteract the damage of trans fats (the type of fat created when unsaturated fats are treated to make them last longer). The low-fat diet combined with the high level of trans fats has made it difficult to achieve the right level of healthy fats in our diets, leading to the development of diseases such as Alzheimer's.

Coconut oil also aids the absorption of vital minerals such as magnesium and calcium, so it can assist in keeping your heart and bones strong and healthy.

In this chapter, we will examine how coconut oil can positively affect some common health conditions.

Why Coconut Oil
Is So Healthy

Coconut oil defies the modern assumption that fatty acids are not good for you. On the contrary, coconut oil is a versatile and effective remedy for a wide range of conditions and also works as a preventative treatment. Whether it is applied topically or consumed, coconut oil can fight unhealthy bacteria and miroorganisms as well as viruses and fungus. It is also extremely beneficial for your brain.

But why? How can coconut oil be so effective in so many ways? In this section we look at how the components of coconut oil help us fight disease and stay strong, healthy, and alert. Then we will look at specific diseases and conditions, so you can see exactly how coconut oil can help you and your loved ones.

Health Benefits of Coconut Oil

antiviral – Coconut oil is made up of medium-chain fatty acids, giving it a deceptively similar structure to viruses. When a virus encounters coconut oil, the virus assumes it is simply bonding with a fellow virus, but once the virus has absorbed the coconut oil, the medium-chain fatty acids destroy the structure of the virus from the inside. The virus disintegrates and becomes harmless without any damage to human tissue.

antimicrobial – Monolaurin is as powerful as bleach at removing unhealthy miroorganisms from the body. However, unlike bleach, monolaurin can differentiate between healthy, vital miroorganisms and unhealthy organisms, so it will only "clean out" those miroorganisms that disrupt the body's equilibrium, providing a healthier balance to the blood stream and digestive tract.

antibacterial – One of the problems with taking prescribed antibiotics is that they tend to destroy healthy bacteria along with the invaders. The lauric acid in coconut oil will destroy lipid-coated "invasive" bacteria, although it allows the probiotics to thrive. Probiotics are not lipid-coated, which is how lauric acid and monolaurin can identify invaders from the healthy probiotic community. Coconut oil is an effective antibacterial whether it is taken internally or applied externally.

antifungal – The three fatty acids in coconut oil—caprylic acid, capric acid, and lauric acid—can all fight yeast, which is the base of a fungal infection. In fact, caprylic acid supplements are sold as commercial antifungal treatments. But why buy a pill if you can take your medication straight from nature?

fuel – When you hear the term "fatty acids," you probably concentrate on that fatal first syllable—*fat*. But the fatty acids in coconut oil are not stored by the human body as fat. Rather, they are converted into an important energy source, called *ketones*, which are vital for the repair and maintenance of bone tissue and brain cells.

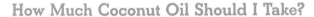

How Much Coconut Oil Should I Take?

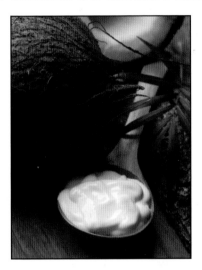

If you want to start taking coconut oil every day for your general health and well-being, your daily dose is determined by your weight. Check out our cooking section to discover innovative ways to incorporate your daily dose into your diet. Or you can simply eat it straight from the spoon!

Weight in lb/kg	Daily dose of virgin coconut oil
25–49 lb/11–22 kg	1 tablespoon
50–74 lb/23–33 kg	1½ tablespoons
75–99 lb/34–44 kg	2 tablespoons
100–124 lb/45–57 kg	2½ tablespoons
125–149 lb/58–66 kg	3 tablespoons
150–174 lb/67–78 kg	3½ tablespoons
175 lb and over/79 kg and over	¼ cup

Losing Weight with Coconut Oil

We know that coconut oil is a medium-chain fatty acid, and you might think that consuming a fat will make you fat. But this is not actually true. During the 1940s, farmers fed coconut oil to their cows, assuming the cows would fatten up—but the opposite happened! The cows became lean and energetic. When the farmers switched to an unsaturated fat, they managed to fatten up their cattle.

All the foods you consume are either released as energy to help you grow new cells, restore damaged cells, and remain active, or they are stored as fat. Naturally, foods with a high nutrient level are more likely to be released as energy, while foods that are difficult to process and digest, and have fewer useful nutrients, will be stored as fat.

The medium-chain triglycerides (or fatty acids) in coconut oil are more water soluble than other fats so they reach the liver faster and are broken down and converted into energy more rapidly. Not only do they convert into energy, but all this extra energy helps you burn off more fat, simply because you are more active! A study by the *International Journal of Obesity and Metabolic Disorders* found that medium-chain triglycerides increase fat burning and calorie expenditure while decreasing your stores of body fat.

Coconut oil also contributes to weight loss by making you less vulnerable to cravings in two ways: First, it helps you digest your food more slowly so you feel full longer; and second, it keeps your sugar levels balanced so you no longer have that "3 p.m. crash" when you energy drops and you crave a sugar rush to boost your energy up. Coconut oil prompts carbohydrates to convert more slowly into glucose after each meal. Your energy is released more consistently, so you stay active for longer periods of time, and there is less excess energy being converted into fat cells.

Coconut Oil Diet Tips

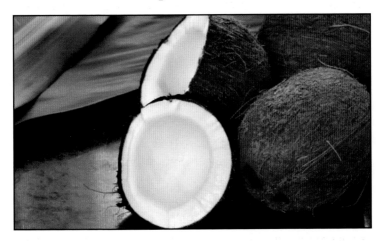

Naturally, coconut oil is a more effective weight-loss remedy when teamed with regular portions of fresh, nutritious food. When cooking, always use virgin coconut oil.

The simplest way to incorporate coconut oil into your diet plan is to stir 1–2 tablespoons of coconut oil into a mug of hot water twenty minutes before every meal. Allow the coconut oil to melt in the water, and then drink it down. Alternately, you could make a nutritious smoothie or even a meal with coconut oil as one of the ingredients! Check out our recipe section for more ideas.

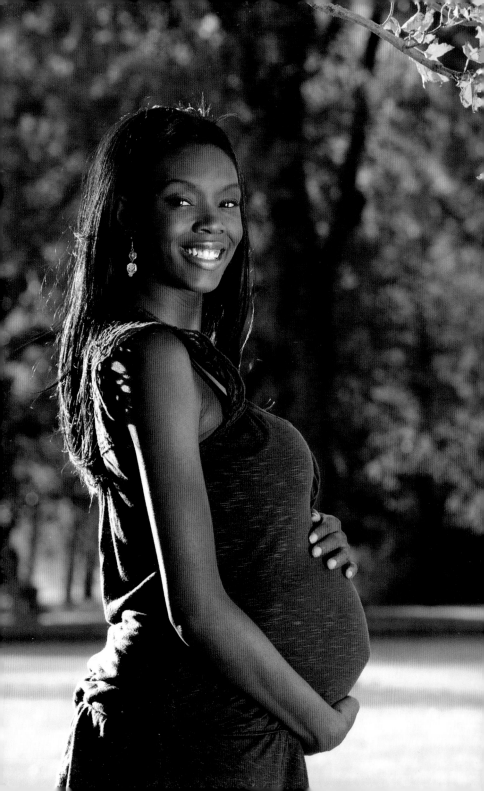

Coconut Oil and Your Health

Coconut Oil During Pregnancy and Infancy

A daily dose of coconut oil is beneficial during pregnancy, as the natural fats help your unborn baby grow and absorb all the essential nutrients. It will also boost your calcium intake by improving your absorption.

You can use coconut oil topically on your stomach to prevent stretch marks. To prepare for labor, you can massage the oil into the perineum—this will strengthen the delicate tissues so they will stretch more easily during child birth.

After the birth, coconut oil on the perineum will help you heal faster. Continue taking a daily dose of three or four tablespoons of coconut oil to increase your milk supply, and you can also massage it into your nipples to prevent cracking.

If your newborn baby suffers from cradle cap, gently massage a small amount of coconut oil into the scalp, then after a few minutes wash the oil off with warm water. You can also use coconut oil as a gentle and natural remedy for diaper rash.

Coconut Oil and Thrush

The high content of lauric acid and caprylic acid make coconut oil an excellent treatment for fungal infections such as thrush or Candida. Both these acids have antibacterial, antifungal, and antimicrobial properties, making them ideal for fighting fungal overgrowth while balancing your bacteria level and fighting infection.

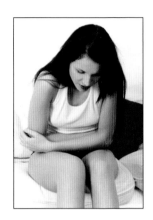

Taking coconut oil treats the cause of Candida rather than simply treating the symptoms, so you can balance your system in the long term and eliminate the distressing side effects of a Candida infection, such as fatigue, mood swings, and abdominal pain. Start by taking one tablespoon a day, and then gradually increase the dose to up to three tablespoons a day. For fungal infections such as athlete's foot, apply coconut oil directly to the afflicted area.

Coconut Oil for Colds and Flu

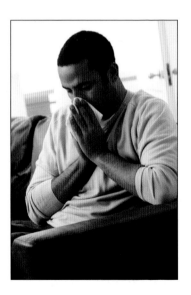

The antiviral properties of coconut oil mean it is an excellent natural treatment for colds and related conditions. Consume between one and three tablespoons a day to boost your immunity.

If you are feeling congested, try combining solid coconut oil with a few drops of essential oil and apply the mixture to your chest. When you have a headache or feel feverish, try massaging plain coconut oil into your temples. A dollop of coconut oil in a cup of hot tea will soothe and heal a sore throat.

A daily dose of coconut oil is also soothing and beneficial for a cough as the oil will destroy the bacteria causing the cough. Try stirring the coconut oil into a cup of hot tea for soothing and therapeutic refreshment.

Coconut Oil and Alzheimer's Disease

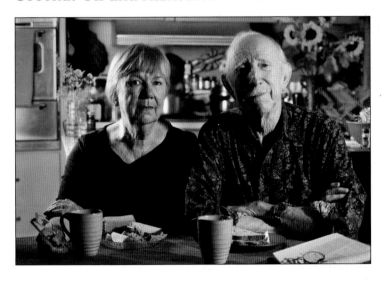

One of the indications of Alzheimer's disease is that some sections of the brain stop processing glucose. For this reason, people with diabetes have a higher risk of developing Alzheimer's disease, as they already have problems processing sugars. Researchers have figured out that, by supplying more energy to the brain, they could find a solution to the downward spiral of Alzheimer's.

The brain uses an energy source called *ketones*. The liver converts medium-chain triglycerides into ketones, and coconut oil is rich in medium-chain triglycerides. Many researchers of small-scale studies have found that daily doses of coconut oil have helped slow the development of Alzheimer's and it is believed this is because the medium-chain triglycerides are providing the necessary energy to keep the brain cells from deteriorating.

Coconut Oil and Crohn's Disease

Crohn's Disease causes major ulcerations along the digestive system, preventing patients from absorbing nutrients and fluids, so they become dehydrated and/or malnourished. Coconut oil works in two ways to ease the symptoms and after-effects of Crohn's disease. First, it helps to heal the ulcerated sections of the digestive tract, and second, it works to increase the absorption of essential nutrients such as 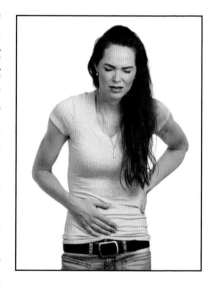 calcium and magnesium. Crohn's patients can also benefit from drinking coconut water, as it is rich in electrolytes, which is lost through malabsorption.

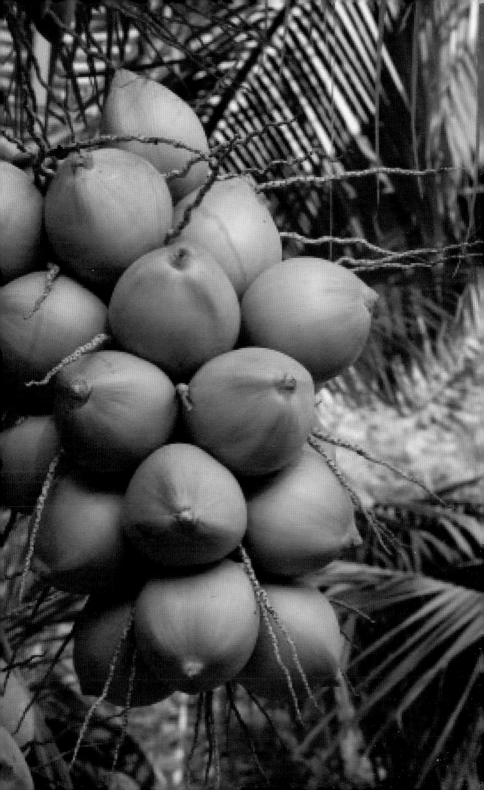

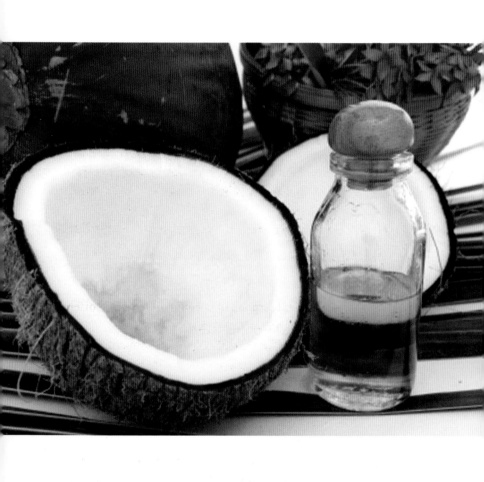

Coconut Oil for Common Ailments

Coconut oil can be beneficial for a wide range of conditions and illnesses. We have listed some of the more common conditions that can be treated with coconut oil either orally or topically. You can also keep coconut oil in your first aid kit as a soothing ointment for rashes and inflammations or as an antibacterial dressing for cuts and scrapes.

Remember, only virgin coconut oil is guaranteed to provide beneficial results.

Ailments to Be Treated with Coconut Oil

acid reflux – Add a tablespoon of coconut oil to tea or coffee up to three times a day for relief of indigestion or reflux.

acne – Coconut oil, applied topically, has excellent short-term and long-term effects for acne sufferers. The antibacterial, antioxidant, and antimicrobial agents clear away the cause of acne while soothing the inflammation and eliminating redness. In the long term, the vitamins E and K in coconut oil will help heal the skin, so there is less scarring.

Apply a small amount to the affected area twice daily until acne disappears. In addition, take a daily dose of coconut oil orally to balance the body's bacteria level and increase the absorption of essential vitamins necessary to keep the skin clear and healthy.

allergies – A daily dose of coconut oil will help relieve allergy symptoms. It will also boost your immune system so you have a stronger resistance to aggravating stimuli.

arthritis – Coconut oil is a powerful anti-inflammatory and it helps increase the absorption of magnesium, an excellent mineral for muscles, joints, and the neurological system. Take a daily oral dose of coconut oil to relieve symptoms both in the short term and the long term.

asthma – Asthma is triggered by inflammation, which usually also limits the absorption of nutrients from food. Coconut oil not only works as an anti-inflammatory, but it also helps increase your ability to absorb nutrients, so you are generally stronger and fitter. The fatty acids in coconut oil are essential for the repair and maintenance of healthy lung tissue. Take a daily dose to counteract asthma symptoms.

athlete's foot – Coconut oil is an antifungal agent so it is an excellent cure for athlete's foot. After showering at night, cover your foot with coconut oil and then place a plastic bag over your foot. Place a sock over the plastic bag to keep the bag in position. Keep the "coconut oil sock" on for at least three hours, preferably all night. In the morning, remove the sock and bag, and wipe your foot dry with a paper towel. Continue this nightly treatment until the fungal infection has disappeared. It should take around five applications to completely eradicate the condition.

cancer – There is a strong scientific argument that cancer is a metabolic disorder, and that cancer cells thrive on glucose and the fermentation of amino acids. However, they cannot produce energy from ketones, the energy source derived from medium-chain acids. In fact, ketones can nurture healthy cells while starving cancer cells. Coconut oil is made up of medium-chain acids that are a natural source of ketones, and the antibiotic and antimicrobial properties of coconut oil can help keep the body strong to fight the debilitating effects of cancer. Take one to three tablespoons of coconut oil every three hours to help fight cancer. For preventative measures, take one standard dose daily.

chicken pox – Chicken pox is caused by an airborne virus that generally lasts a week and is characterized by itchy spots that scab over before falling off. Usually, chicken pox is more irritating than dangerous. Coconut oil has antiviral properties and is particularly soothing, so it is the ideal treatment to keep a patient comfortable during the itchiest days of the illness. Apply coconut oil directly to blistered area. A highly recommended recipe for a soothing cream is a mixture of one tablespoon of coconut oil, one tablespoon of chamomile ointment, and ¼ teaspoon of cayenne pepper.

chronic fatigue – Coconut oil is a great energy booster and the medium-chain fatty acids help fight the infectious organisms believed to trigger chronic fatigue. Take one dose of coconut oil daily to combat the symptoms of chronic fatigue and strengthen the immune system and increase your energy.

cold sores (herpes) – The antiviral properties in coconut oil will help fight the herpes virus that causes cold sores. Apply coconut oil up to three times a day, and take a daily oral dose of coconut oil to prevent or minimize further breakouts.

constipation – Coconut oil is both fibrous and easily absorbed so it is an excellent remedy for constipation. It also works as a cleansing and balancing agent for your entire digestive tract, so regular doses will have a positive effect on your digestion.

corns – Corns are painful cone-shaped lumps of dead skin that accumulate on the feet, usually as a result of pressure from poorly-fitting shoes. You can soften the corn with a nightly application of coconut oil. The best way to remove corns permanently is to start by soaking the feet in a foot bath of warm water with ½ cup sea salt and ½ cup baking soda. After twenty minutes, rub the feet gently with a pumice stone and then apply coconut oil. For best results, cover the foot with a plastic bag and a sock and leave the "coconut sock" on overnight. Repeat nightly until the corn has dissolved.

cuts and abrasions – Coconut oil is an effective natural antibacterial, so a thin layer of coconut oil applied to a wound will be soothing and will destroy any bacteria.

diabetes – Diabetics who cannot control their blood sugar levels can benefit from daily doses of coconut oil. The fatty acids in coconut oil slow down the digestive process, converting the carbohydrates into glucose at a regular rate so the blood sugar levels stay steady.

ear aches – The medium-chain fatty acids in coconut oil will fight both viral infections and bacterial infections, while the warmth of gently heated oil will also be soothing to the painful site. Melt the oil and apply carefully with an eye-dropper. However, seek medical advice before any application if the ear drum is damaged.

eczema – Eczema is characterized by dry, itchy, and inflamed skin. The antibacterial, antifungal, and antimicrobial properties of coconut oil can heal the skin and prevent secondary infection, while the texture of the coconut oil is soothing to the skin. Apply a thin layer to the affected skin daily until the eczema has cleared. A daily dose of coconut oil every day will boost the immune system, helping to heal and prevent further outbreaks of eczema.

foot care – Use coconut oil as massage oil for sore and swollen feet. The oil will also soften dead skin so exfoliation is easier and more effective.

hay fever – Using a cotton swab, apply a light layer of coconut oil inside each nostril. This will prevent pollen from irritating the nasal cavity.

heart disease – The medium-chain fatty acids in coconut oil will increase the healthy cholesterol level in the body, improving your overall health and lowering the risk of heart disease. There is also a proven link between chronic bacterial and viral infections and the development of heart disease. So a daily dose of coconut oil will work to prevent heart disease by moderating your cholesterol level and lowering your risk of infectious illnesses that undermine heart health.

hemorrhoids – Coconut oil is both soothing and clears infection. Dry the afflicted area carefully with a cotton ball and then gently apply a layer of coconut oil. Repeat after each bowel movement.

hives and rashes – Apply a thin layer of coconut oil to the affected area daily until symptoms subside. Additionally, take a daily dose of coconut oil to improve your immune system.

insect bites and stings – Apply a small amount of coconut oil on insect bites to take away the sting and itchiness.

kidney stones – Kidney stones are painful shards of crystallised calcium that become lodged in the urethra. While most people have a chemical in their system to prevent the formation of kidney stones, others have a chronic problem with kidney stones. If you feel the early indications of a kidney stone, make a mixture of equal parts coconut oil and lemon juice (or lime juice, if preferred) and drink this once a day, followed by a large glass of water. This will soften or disintegrate the stone, making it easier to pass out through the urine.

liver – The antimicrobial properties in coconut oil are believed to be extremely beneficial for repairing damage in the liver and removing dangerous microorganisms. Some studies suggest that regular doses of coconut oil could be used as treatment for cirrhosis of the liver.

multiple sclerosis (MS) – Coconut oil improves the absorption of magnesium, an essential mineral for neurological health. The medium-chain fatty acids create ketones, the energy source required by the brain, so that damaged brain cells can be repaired. This in turn can improve the communication between the brain and the rest of the body.

muscle soreness, stiff joints – Coconut oil lubricates muscles and joints by increasing blood circulation. You can take a daily dose of coconut oil to improve your muscle strength and tone, and you can treat painful areas by using warm coconut oil as a massage lotion, to soothe and heal the afflicted area.

poison ivy and poison oak (also nettles) – Poison ivy contains a toxic resin called urushiol that causes an extremely irritating skin inflammation. Massage warm coconut oil into the area to soothe the itchiness and eradicate the toxins.

psoriasis – Psoriasis is a chronic skin condition, causing itchy, scaling skin. Consume two tablespoons of coconut oil a day to improve the condition of the skin and strengthen the immune system. You can also soothe the afflicted area by applying a thin layer of warm coconut oil.

ringworm – As coconut oil has antifungal properties, it is an excellent natural treatment for ringworm, which is an extremely contagious fungal skin infection. Using a cotton ball, gently apply coconut oil to the afflicted area up to three times a day. Be extremely conscientious about hand hygiene, washing your hands before and after applying the oil, as ringworm is contagious.

sinusitis – The nasal congestion characteristic of sinusitis is caused by the inflammation of blood vessels to the point where nasal tissues become swollen. This swelling can be the result of a bacterial or viral infection, so coconut oil is an ideal natural remedy for eliminating the source of infection. Take a daily dose of coconut oil to fight the virus or bacteria.

sunburn and windburn – Coconut oil can stimulate the renewal of cell growth, and this is particularly necessary when the skin cells have been damaged by the elements. Apply a thin layer of coconut oil to the areas on the body that are affected by sunburn or windburn. Reapply when needed until symptoms disappear.

thyroid – An underactive thyroid lowers your body temperature so you always feel cold, particularly in your hands and feet. While most other oils are detrimental to people with an under-active thyroid, the medium-chain fatty acids in coconut oil will boost your metabolism and raise your basal body temperature so your thyroid will perform more efficiently.

ulcers – Ulcers are small, painful holes in the digestive tract that can affect your appetite and your overall digestion. Coconut oil is an excellent long-term natural remedy for ulcers, as it kills the bacteria causing the ulcer. Start a routine of a daily dose of coconut oil to treat and eliminate ulcers.

urinary tract infection – A UTI is characterized by frequent, painful urination and can be associated with fever, nausea, or bleeding. It is important to treat a UTI promptly to prevent the infection traveling into the kidneys. Coconut oil is an excellent natural remedy, particularly when combined with coconut water. The coconut oil will kill the bacteria and soothe the urinary tract. The coconut water assists in soothing and healing the urinary tract, while ensuring you retain the right level of electrolytes. Take three doses of coconut oil daily, and drink three generous glasses of warm water with coconut oil throughout the day.

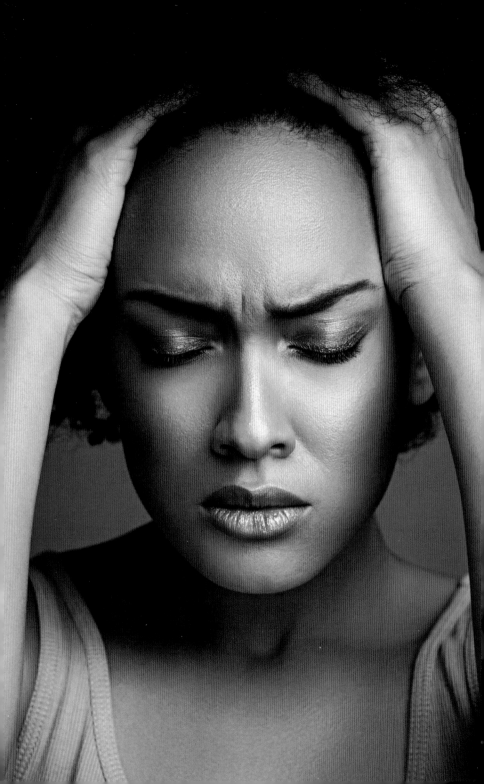

Possible Negative Effects of Coconut Oil

It is possible that you may feel some negative physical effects when you first start taking coconut oil regularly. There are two possible reasons for this—either you are having an allergic response or a detoxifying response.

If you are allergic to coconut oil, you may experience a cough, a rash, hives, or swelling in your face, eyelids, throat, tongue, and eyes. If you experience any of these symptoms, stop taking coconut oil until you can establish exactly what has caused the allergic reaction. Seek medical attention immediately if these symptoms appear suddenly or severely.

However, other symptoms may simply be your body's reaction to the detoxifying effects of coconut oil. Since coconut oil works as an antiviral and antifungal agent, you may feel feverish and/or flu-like symptoms after taking it for a few days. You may also experience some nausea, gas, and/or soft stools. These symptoms are caused by the release of toxins into your blood stream in response to the cleansing power of coconut oil. Drink plenty of water to help flush out the toxins and cut down on your dose of coconut oil if you experience vomiting or diarrhea.

If the symptoms are mild, try lowering the dose or incorporating the coconut oil into food rather than eating it undiluted.

In time, these symptoms will subside and you will start to feel the amazing effects of this wonderful oil!

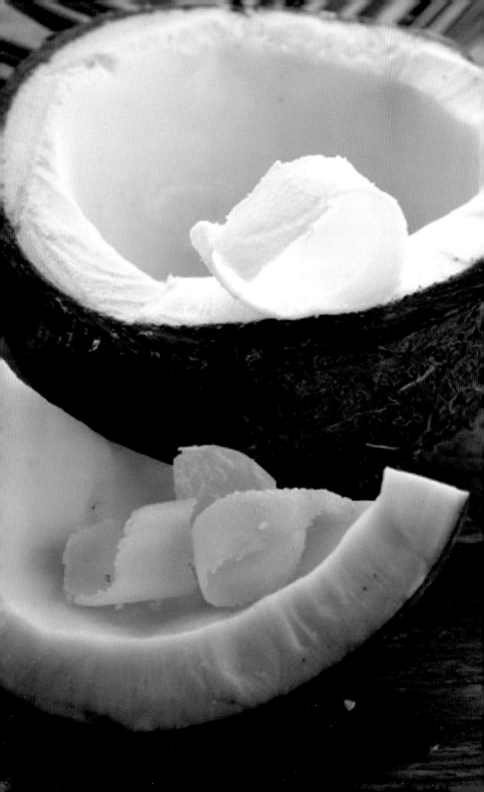

Coconut Oil Recipes

After reading about the health benefits of coconut oil, you might be wondering how to incorporate sufficient coconut oil into your diet. The good news is that you have countless options besides swallowing a spoonful of straight coconut oil three times a day. Not only can you use coconut oil as your cooking oil, there are also countless delicious and nutritious recipes that incorporate it.

Note: The coconut butter mentioned in some recipes refers to organic whole coconut meat in concentrated form. It is also known as coconut cream concentrate and is generally watered down in recipes. Coconut milk works as a substitute for coconut butter if you eliminate some of the fluid content from the recipe.

Beverages
Coconut oil can be a natural addition to your favorite daily beverage, whether it is adding some cream to your cup of coffee or a new take on hot chocolate!

Coconut Cocoa

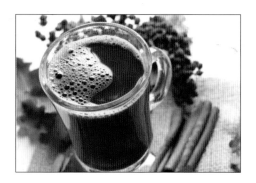

Ingredients:

    1 tablespoon melted virgin coconut oil
    1 tablespoon cocoa powder
    Pinch Himalayan salt
    ¼ teaspoon organic whole sugar (minimum)
    ¾ cup boiling water

To melt the coconut oil, swill boiling water around a mug to heat it, and then tip out the water. Swill the virgin coconut oil around in the mug and it will melt quickly. Stir in the cocoa powder and salt. Add sweetener of choice, then pour boiling water into the cup. Stir and add cream or milk to taste.

Dairy-Free Coffee Creamer

This delicious creamer will lighten your coffee and tea while providing your daily dose of nutritious coconut oil.

Ingredients:

    1 cup cashew nuts, soaked overnight, rinsed
    ¼ cup honey
    ½ teaspoon vanilla extract
    ½ cup coconut milk
    2 tablespoons coconut oil, melted

Place cashews, honey, vanilla, and coconut milk in a blender. Blend until smooth and creamy, while pouring a steady drizzle of coconut oil into the mix.

    The coffee creamer can be stored in the refrigerator for up to a week.

Coconut Latte

Ingredients:

    1–2 tablespoons coconut butter
    1–3 tablespoons coconut oil
    ⅔ cup whole milk
    1 cup espresso
    2 tablespoons coconut flavored syrup

Brew espresso and add coconut butter. Pour into cups.

    Using an espresso steamer, steam the milk and coconut oil and add to the cups of espresso.

Iced Coconut Mochaccino

Ingredients:

    ¾ cup cold, strong coffee (partly frozen if desired)
    ½ cup organic coconut milk

2 tablespoons fudge sauce, cold
2–4 ice cubes
1 tablespoon coconut oil, melted

Place all ingredients except coconut oil in a blender and blend until well combined, pouring coconut oil into the cappuccino in a steady stream. Top with freshly whipped cream.

Hot Fudge Sauce

Ingredients:
    ¾ cup sugar
    ½ cup cocoa powder
    ¾ cup heavy cream
    4 tablespoons butter
    1–2 tablespoons coconut oil
    1½ teaspoons vanilla extract

Combine all ingredients except vanilla extract in a saucepan over medium heat.

When butter is melted, increase the heat and bring fudge to a boil, whisking constantly. Boil for 1 minute. Remove from heat and stir in vanilla.

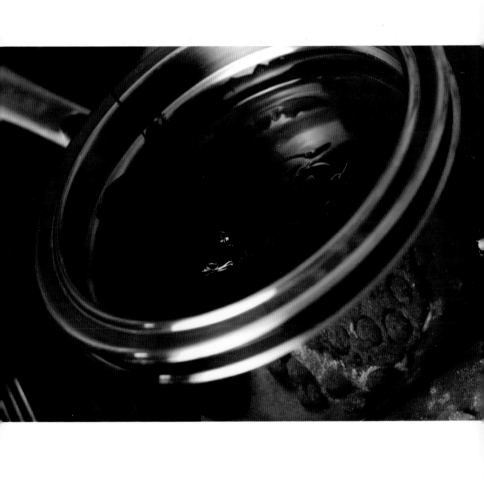

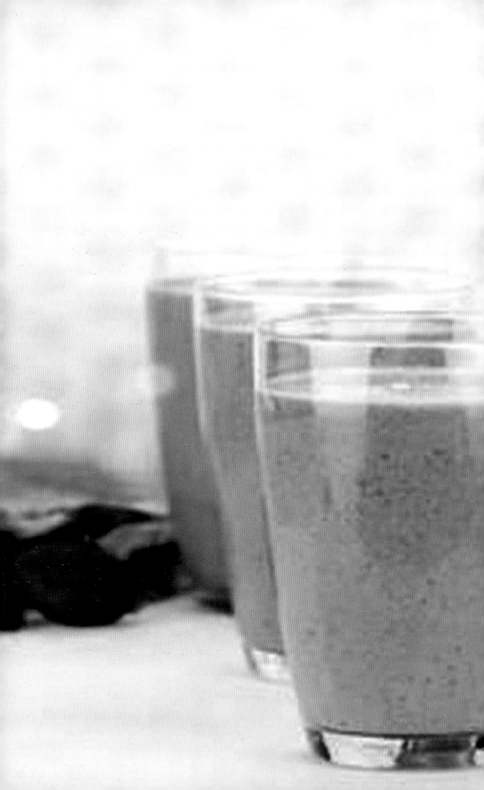

Smoothies

These delicious smoothies will provide you with all the energy and nutrients you need for an optimum start to your day. Best of all, the coconut oil will help you absorb a greater level of vitamins and minerals, as well as soothing your digestive tract.

Green Coconut Dream
Serves 3–6

Ingredients:

3 cold, organic granny smith apples, sliced or diced
½ cucumber, thinly chopped
3 tablespoons coconut oil
1 cup coconut water
1 cup apple juice
1 avocado, pitted
1 cup fresh organic spinach leaves
1 cup chopped pineapple
1 cup crushed ice

Place the apples, cucumber, spinach, and avocado in the blender with the apple juice. Blend until smooth.

Add ½ cup crushed ice and pineapple, blend well. Add coconut oil, coconut water, and the rest of the crushed ice. Serve chilled with fresh mint.

Mixed Berry Smoothie

Blend the following ingredients in a blender:

1 cup of frozen mixed berries: blueberries, strawberries, raspberries

½ frozen banana

½ cup coconut milk

¼ cup orange juice

½ cup water

3 tablespoons protein powder (optional)

3–4 tablespoons virgin coconut oil, melted

3–4 ice cubes

Coconut Cream Smoothie

Ingredients:

1½ cups coconut milk

5 large eggs

2 tablespoons virgin coconut oil, melted

2 tablespoons coconut butter, softened

½ teaspoon nutmeg

½ teaspoon ground ginger

½ teaspoon cinnamon

¼ teaspoon sea salt

4 or 5 frozen ripe bananas

Blend all the ingredients except the bananas, until thoroughly mixed. Add the bananas and blend until smooth. Serve with nutmeg sprinkled on top.

Banana Coconut Smoothie

Serves 2–4

Ingredients:

2 frozen bananas

2 tablespoons virgin coconut oil

½ cup almond/coconut milk

1 teaspoon vanilla extract

½ cup crushed ice

Place the bananas, vanilla, and almond milk/coconut milk in the blender. Blend until smooth.

Add the crushed ice, followed by the coconut oil. Be sure to blend it fully to avoid chunks of ice or coconut oil.

Serve immediately.

Coconut Orange Vitamin Kick

Serves 1–3

Ingredients:

3 full oranges, peeled, chopped, seeds removed

2 full peaches, pitted

4 tablespoons coconut oil

¼ cup shredded coconut

1 cup organic orange juice, chilled

½ cup crushed ice

Add orange juice, oranges, and peaches. Blend until smooth.

Slowly add the crushed ice, shredded coconut, and coconut oil; these will take some time to fully blend into the current mixture.

Serve as cold as possible.

Coconut Strawberry Smoothie

Serves 1–3

Ingredients:

    10–15 frozen strawberries
    ½ cup full fat natural yogurt or coconut milk yogurt
    3 tablespoons virgin coconut oil
    1 cup coconut milk
    ⅓ cup crushed ice

Place the yogurt and coconut oil in the blender first. Add a couple strawberries at a time, blending until smooth between each addition. Add the coconut milk, especially if and when the blending becomes difficult. Add crushed ice until completely smooth.
    Serve immediately.

Coconut Berry Freeze

Serves 2

Ingredients:

    1 cup blueberries
    1 cup acai berries
    1 cup strawberries
    ¼ cup raspberries
    3 tablespoons coconut oil
    1 cup almond milk
    1 cup crushed ice

Place the berries and almond milk in the blender. These ingredients are plentiful, so cut the recipe in half if necessary. Blend until smooth.

Add coconut oil followed by crushed ice. Blend until smooth.
Serve while cold.

Banana Orange Smoothie

Blend the following ingredients in a blender:
1 banana
6 strawberries
½ cup orange juice
3 tablespoons virgin coconut oil (liquefied)
1 tablespoon coconut butter
3 tablespoons Greek yogurt
3 ice cubes

Banana Oat Smoothie

Blend the following ingredients in a blender:
2 frozen bananas
½ cup rolled oat flakes
1 cup milk (use more or less to adjust to desired
consistency)
½ cup peanut butter
1–2 tablespoons coconut oil, melted
Dash cinnamon
1 teaspoon vanilla

Apricot Coconut Smoothie

Blend the following ingredients in the blender:
1½ cups coconut milk
4 egg yolks
1 tablespoon virgin coconut oil, melted

2 tablespoons coconut flakes
2 tablespoons honey
¾ cup frozen apricots
½ cup frozen pineapple
1 teaspoon vanilla extract
Dash of salt

Rum Piña Colada

Ingredients:

½ cup diced pineapple
3 tablespoons virgin coconut oil
4 cherries (to taste)
2 bananas
1 cup crushed ice
½ cup good-quality white rum

Place all of the fruit and the rum in a blender, and blend until smooth.

Add the coconut oil, followed by the crushed ice, and blend until smooth being sure to blend the oil in thoroughly. Serve in chilled glasses.

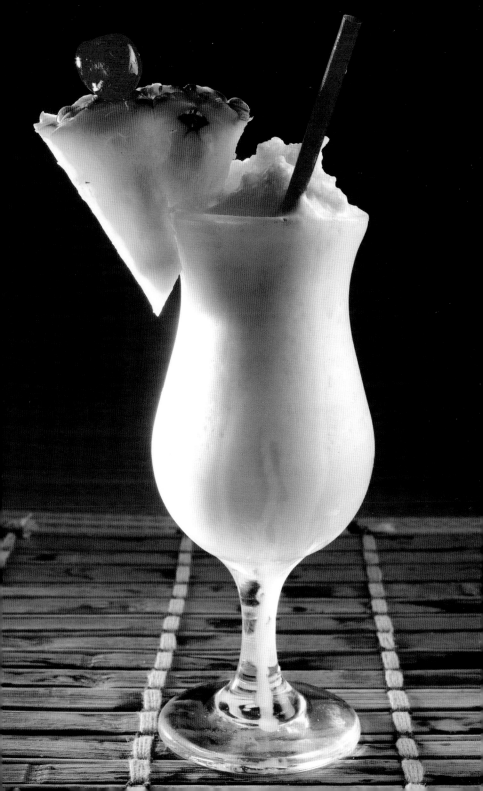

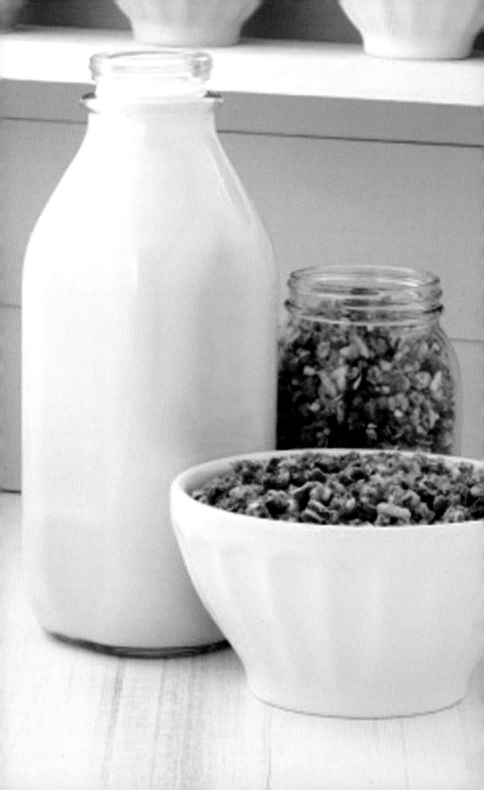

Breakfast Recipes

Buckwheat Granola with Coconut Oil, Cherries, and Cacao

This granola is simple to make and packs a nutritional punch with lots of superfoods.

Ingredients:

1 cup buckwheat groats, soaked
¼ cup almonds
¼ cup cashews
3 tablespoons raw honey
2 tablespoons expeller-pressed coconut oil
1 teaspoon cinnamon, ground
¼ cup organic cherries, dried
¼ cup pumpkin seeds
2 tablespoons organic raw cacao nibs
1 tablespoon coconut, shredded
Non-dairy milk, as desired

Place buckwheat groats in a large bowl.

Process almonds and cashews in a food processor until they resemble coarse crumbs.

Add almond and cashew mixture to buckwheat groats, along with other ingredients, except milk. Stir to combine.

Place mixture on a dehydrator tray and dehydrate for about four hours, or until dried. You may also heat on a low temperature (150°F/65°C) in an oven for about thirty minutes, or until dried.

Quinoa Porridge with Coconut Oil and Cinnamon
Serves 2

Ingredients
1 cup quinoa
½ teaspoons Celtic sea salt
1 teaspoon cinnamon
2 tablespoons of organic maple syrup
1 tablespoon coconut oil
Almond milk to serve

Bring 2 cups of water to a boil in a wide saucepan. Add quinoa, Celtic sea salt, cinnamon, maple syrup, and coconut oil. Cover and reduce heat and simmer for twelve minutes.Remove from heat and scoop into a bowl add almond milk and enjoy.

Coconut French Toast
Serves 2–4

Ingredients:
3 organic free-range eggs
½ cup rapadura
½ cup almond milk
⅓ teaspoon baking soda

2 tablespoons coconut oil
Cinnamon for dusting
2 slices sourdough bread per person

Option One

Mix eggs with almond milk, baking soda, and coconut oil. Pour mixture over bread and refrigerate 2–4 hours.

Place in oven at 450°F (232°C) for twenty-five to thirty minutes. Top with a mix of cinnamon and rapadura.

Option Two

Mix eggs with almond milk, baking soda, and coconut oil. Soak bread in mixture and place a single piece in a heated frying pan with ¼ cup coconut oil.

Fry until golden brown, top with a mix of cinnamon and rapadura.

Cheesy Bacon Muffins

Ingredients:

6 strips bacon
3 eggs
¼ teaspoon salt
3 tablespoons coconut flour
¼ teaspoon baking powder
4 oz (115 g) cheddar cheese, shredded/diced
Coconut oil (for greasing muffin tin)

Preheat oven to 400°F (205°C). Fry bacon in a frying pan until crispy. Set aside and save the bacon drippings.

Blend eggs, 2 tablespoons of bacon drippings, and salt in a mixing bowl.

Add coconut flour and baking powder. Mix thoroughly until there are no lumps.

Crumble bacon and add to batter along with cheese. Mix until well combined.

Grease your muffin tin with coconut oil.

Pour batter into muffin tin and bake for fifteen minutes.

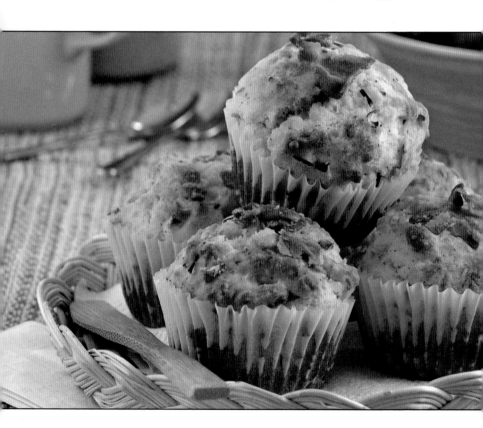

Harvest Fruits with Cashew Butter and Coconut Oil

Serves 4

Ingredients:

    1 juicy pear, cored
    1 juicy apple, cored
    1 tablespoons chia seeds
    3 dates
    3 tablespoons cashews
    1 teaspoons vanilla
    ½ teaspoon Himalayan sea salt
    Coconut water, to thin
    2 tablespoons melted coconut oil
    1 pear, cut into chunks
    1 red apple, cut into chunks
    1 green apple, cut into chunks
    1 Asian pear, cut into chunks
    Shredded coconut for garnish

Place juicy pear and juicy apple in a blender and blend until smooth. Add chia seeds, dates, and cashews and pulse twice to combine. Let sit for at least ten minutes. Add vanilla and sea salt and blend again till smooth (you may need to add coconut water to combine the ingredients). With the blender running, drizzle in oil and continue blending until emulsified. Divide fruit among four bowls and top each with a large dollop of the cashew butter. Sprinkle with shredded coconut.

French Banana Toast

Serves 4
Preparation Time: 10 minutes

Ingredients:

1 banana
1 cup milk
1 cup coconut milk
1 teaspoon vanilla
¼ teaspoon nutmeg
¼ teaspoon cinnamon
1 ½ teaspoons cornstarch
¼ teaspoon salt
12+ slices bread
Coconut oil

Heat a frying pan and add coconut oil. Blend banana, milk, coconut milk, vanilla, spices, and cornstarch in a blender until smooth. Pour into a shallow dish. Coat each slice of bread with the mixture and place in the pan.

Cook until golden brown and then flip over to cook other side. Serve with maple syrup.

Apple Cinnamon Pancakes

Ingredients:

1 cup whole wheat pastry flour
1 teaspoon baking powder
¼ teaspoon baking soda
½ teaspoon salt

⅛ teaspoon cinnamon
4 eggs
1 cup whole milk plain yogurt
¼ cup milk
¼ cup chopped walnuts
¼ cup shredded coconut
¼ cup apple topping (recipe below)
Coconut oil

Apple Topping

4 medium sized Fuji apples, diced small, but not fine
1–2 tablespoons whole sugar, as desired
⅛ –¼ teaspoons cinnamon, to taste
½ teaspoon vanilla
1 tablespoon water
1 tablespoon butter

Topping: In a small saucepan, combine apples, sugar, cinnamon, and vanilla. Set aside ¼ cup of the raw apple mixture, and add water and butter to the rest and simmer on low heat while you make the pancakes, stirring occasionally. Do not boil. The apples are ready when they are soft but still firm and aromatic.

Pancakes: Sift together flour, baking powder, soda, salt, and cinnamon.

In a separate bowl, beat eggs, then blend in yogurt and milk until smooth. Add egg mixture to dry ingredients, stirring only until moistened. The batter does not need to be completely smooth and should still be lumpy. Add the extra apples, the walnuts, and coconut and gently stir to combine.

Preheat a frying pan to medium-low heat and grease lightly with coconut oil. Ladle batter to the desired pancake size, spreading it gently and evenly to about ⅓-inch thick. When tops start to bubble, flip to cook the other side. Flip only once and do not press or otherwise disturb while cooking. Re-grease pan with more coconut oil as needed.

Serve with maple syrup, coconut shreds, and/or stewed apples.

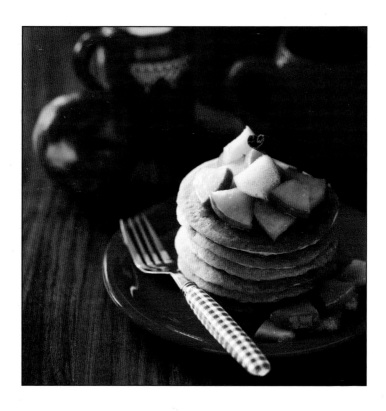

Chocolate Hazelnut Spread

Ingredients:

2 cups hazelnuts

½ cup dark chocolate, cut into chunks

½ cup powdered sugar or honey

55 g cocoa powder

1 tablespoon virgin coconut oil

½ teaspoon vanilla extract

½ teaspoon salt

Preheat oven to 355°F (180°C).

Place the hazelnuts on a cookie sheet in a single layer. Roast the nuts for fifteen minutes.

Meanwhile, melt chocolate with coconut oil in the top of a double boiler.

When nuts are done, place them between paper towels and rub to remove skins.

Place all ingredients in a food processor and blend until smooth.

Store in an airtight container, either in the fridge or pantry, depending on the consistency you desire.

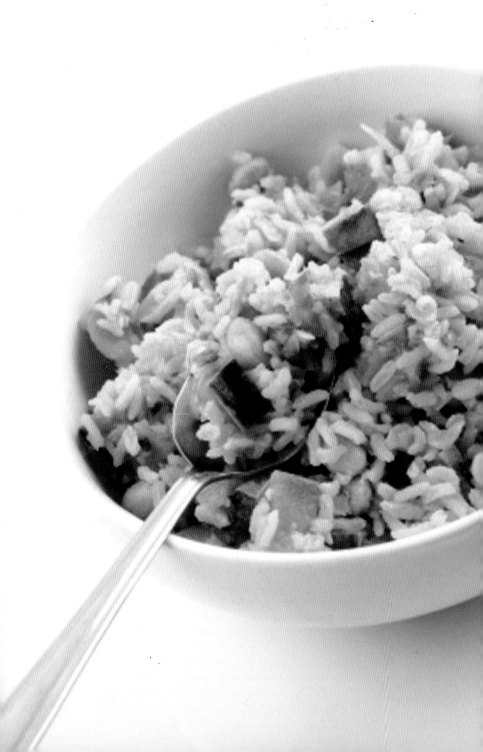

Lunch Recipes

Potatoes and Green Peas in Pumpkin Sauce with Coconut-Lime Rice

Ingredients:

2 tablespoons coconut oil
1 tablespoons olive oil
1 Vidalia onion, sliced
Himalayan sea salt, to taste
2 garlic cloves, minced
White pepper, to taste
2 potatoes, diced
1½ cups water or coconut water
1-inch piece ginger, minced
2 teaspoons turmeric
2 teaspoons coriander
1 teaspoons cumin
1 or 2 teaspoons chili powder
1 cup puréed pumpkin
1½ cups green peas
1 tomato, diced
½ cup plain coconut or almond yogurt
2 tablespoons coconut oil
2 cups cooked basmati rice

½ cup coconut milk
Zest of 1 lime

Heat the oils in a large saucepan over low-medium heat. Add the
onion, season with salt, and cook for about ten minutes to lightly
caramelize the onions. Add the garlic and cook for one minute.
Season with salt and pepper, then add the potatoes, 1½ cups water
(to start), ginger, and spices. Cover and cook about ten minutes,
stirring occasionally and adding more water if needed. Stir in
the pumpkin, peas, tomato, yogurt, and coconut oil and cook for
a minute or two to heat through. Remove from the heat. Combine
the rice, coconut milk, and lime zest in a bowl. Divide the rice
among four plates and top with the potatoes and peas.

Makes 4 servings

Savory Corn Cakes

Ingredients:

1 cup fresh sweet corn (corn cut from 2 ears of corn)
¼ cup chives, garlic chives, or small green onions, chopped
2 eggs
2 tablespoons virgin coconut oil, melted
¼ cup coconut flour
¼ cup fine cornmeal
½ teaspoon salt
¼ teaspoon black pepper
2 tablespoons olive oil, coconut oil, or butter

Purée ¾ of the corn and chives in a mixer. Place into a bowl, add
eggs and 2 tablespoons coconut oil. Mix well. Add coconut flour,
cornmeal, salt, and pepper. Mix gently until well combined.

Heat additional oil in frying pan over medium-low heat. Place large spoonfuls of batter into the pan, flatten gently, and cook until golden brown. Flip and cook other side. Serve with sour cream and chutney.

Asian Broccoli Salad with Coconut Oil

Ingredients:

1 cup broccoli florets
¼ cup almonds, sliced
¼ cup currants or organic golden raisins
¼ cup of a Habanera pepper
¼ teaspoon fresh garlic, minced
2 tablespoons expeller-pressed coconut oil
¼ of an avocado
1 teaspoon tahini
1 teaspoon lemon juice
Pinch of sea salt

Steam broccoli florets for approximately ten minutes, until slightly tender but not overcooked.

Place in a large bowl and stir in almonds and currants or raisins. In a blender, mix pepper, garlic, coconut oil, avocado, lemon juice, tahini, and salt until smooth.

Pour avocado mixture over broccoli and stir completely, coating the broccoli. Serve immediately in individual bowls.

Garlic Chicken Bites

Ingredients:

2 lbs (1 kg) ground chicken

½ teaspoon garlic powder
½ teaspoon onion powder
1 teaspoon crushed red pepper flakes
2 teaspoon chili powder
1 teaspoon salt
Fresh ground pepper
2 eggs
1 cup breadcrumbs
Coconut oil, as needed

Mix all ingredients except coconut oil together until well blended. Add more breadcrumbs if mixture looks too sticky.

Heat coconut oil in a pan over medium heat and drop chicken mixture into pan, shaping into nuggets. Cook until golden brown on both sides and serve.

Chicken and Coconut Rice

Ingredients:

1 cup white rice, al dente, or lightly cooked
¼ cup shredded coconut
2 tablespoons coconut oil
⅓ cup chopped pineapple
⅓ cup chopped red onion
2 tablespoons lemon juice
1 chicken breast, chopped

Heat a frying pan and add the rice and chicken. Cook for fifteen minutes. Be careful not to burn the rice.

When the rice and chicken are thoroughly cooked, add the coconut oil and shredded coconut. Simmer for three to six minutes. Add the lemon juice, chopped pineapple, and red onion to the skillet. Continue to simmer for up to ten minutes. The ingredients will be fully cooked when the smell of the dish becomes rich and heavy.

Coconut Pasta Salad

Serves 1–2

Ingredients:

1 cup spelt pasta, cooked
½ cup chopped onions (red, traditional, sweet, or mixed)
¼ cup chopped carrots
¼ cup chopped celery
3 tablespoons coconut oil
⅓ cup coconut shavings, organic and fresh
¼ cup raspberry vinaigrette dressing

Lightly mix the spelt pasta with the raspberry vinaigrette dressing. The dressing should mix with any leftover water that was not fully strained from the pasta.

Gently mix in the coconut oil thoroughly, followed by the shavings and the onions.

Top the dish with the carrots and celery; they can also be mixed in with the whole salad.

Serve cold.

Coconut Chicken Satay

Serves 12

Ingredients:

1½ lbs (750 g) frozen boneless, skinless chicken thighs,
Thawed wooden or bamboo skewers

Marinade:

1 small onion, chopped
3 cloves garlic, chopped
⅛ teaspoon ground ginger
½ teaspoon dried turmeric
2 teaspoons cumin
1 teaspoon red pepper flakes
¼ cup oyster sauce or fish sauce
⅓ cup brown sugar
2 tablespoons vegetable oil

Coconut Peanut Sauce

1 cup coconut peanut butter
⅛ cup soy sauce
½ teaspoon red pepper flakes
2 tablespoons brown sugar
2 teaspoons lime juice
½ cup hot water
⅛ cup oyster sauce
⅓ cup coconut butter
2 teaspoons sesame oil

Marinade:

Blend all ingredients on high heat for two minutes. Pour into a sealed marinating dish with the chicken. Marinate for several hours, stirring periodically to coat chicken thoroughly. Cut marinated chicken into 2-inch (5 cm) cubes. Soak bamboo skewers in water for twenty minutes so they don't burn while cooking. Thread chicken onto skewers, and it's ready to grill.

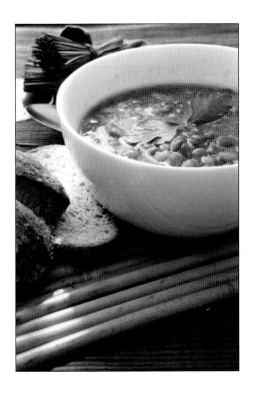

Coconut Peanut Sauce

Blend all ingredients on high heat. Serve with chicken skewers.

Soups

Delicious and nutritious, these heart-warming soups will fill you with energy and well-being.

Creamy Lentil Soup

Ingredients:

1½ cups lentils, soaked
2 tablespoons apple cider vinegar
1 quart chicken stock
2 cups coconut milk
2 tablespoons coconut oil
1 large sweet onion, chopped
1 tablespoon garlic crushed
1–3 tablespoons fresh ginger, minced
½ teaspoon–1 tablespoon crushed red chili flakes
1 teaspoon cumin
1 teaspoon coriander
¼ teaspoon salt
1 organic yellow pepper, chopped
1 organic orange pepper, chopped
1 organic red pepper, chopped
1 quart diced tomatoes
1 cup tomato juice
1 lemon, juiced

Soak lentils in warm water mixed with apple cider vinegar for six hours, and then drain well.

Place lentils in a large pot and cover with 4 inches (10 cm) of water. Bring to a boil, then lower temperature and simmer for thirty minutes. Skim off any foam that rises to the top. Remove from heat and drain well.

Return the lentils to the soup pot along with chicken stock, coconut milk, coconut oil, onion, garlic, ginger, and spices. Simmer for one hour, stirring occasionally, then add the peppers, tomatoes, and tomato juice. Cook for two hours, or until lentils are tender. Remove from heat and stir in lemon juice.

Coconut Bean Soup

Serves 4–6

Ingredients:

4 cups warm water
¼ cup pure organic coconut milk
3 tablespoons virgin coconut oil
½ cup fresh unmodified pinto beans
¼ cup fresh and natural chickpeas
½ cup organic green beans
1 cup raw (not frozen) organic broccoli
½ cup carrots, diced

Pour the warm water in a large pot and turn the stove on low heat. Add the broccoli and carrots. Leave this on the stove while keeping an eye on it for about forty-five minutes.

Add the coconut milk, coconut oil, and green beans to the soup. Turn the heat up by a small increment and mix the soup. Wait about twenty minutes and add the beans and chickpeas.

After letting the full mixture cook until the aroma is enticing, add desired seasonings and herbs. When the fully mixed contents of the pot come to a simmer, the dish is done cooking. Turn the stove off and let cool for five minutes. Serve in bowls, preferably with salad and/or fresh sourdough bread.

Pumpkin Curry Soup

Ingredients:
- ¼ cup coconut oil
- 1 onion, diced
- 2 lbs (1 kg) chopped pumpkin
- 1½ quarts chicken stock
- 2 cloves garlic, pressed
- 2 teaspoon salt

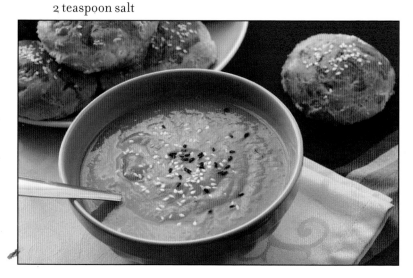

¼ teaspoon crushed red pepper flakes or to taste
1+ tablespoon curry powder
1 teaspoon coriander
Pinch cayenne pepper
2 cups coconut milk

Heat the oil in saucepan and cook onions and garlic until soft.
Add pumpkin, stock, salt, and spices.
Bring to a boil, then simmer for twenty minutes.
Allow to cool, then blend the soup in batches in a food processor. Return to gentle heat and stir in coconut milk. Taste to check if it is spicy enough. If not, add more spices to taste.
Serve sprinkled with nutmeg and with a side dish of crusty bread.

Roasted Cauliflower and Bacon Soup

Ingredients:

1 head cauliflower, cut into pieces
¼ cup coconut oil
Salt and pepper
2–3 pieces bacon, diced
¼–½ cup white onion, diced
2 garlic cloves, minced
1 teaspoon fresh thyme
7 oz (200 g) mushrooms, sliced
¼ cup white wine
3 cups chicken broth
¾ cup full fat coconut milk
2 tablespoons butter

Preheat oven to 400°F (205°C).

Use 2 tablespoons of the coconut oil to coat the coconut pieces. Roast the coconut pieces for twenty-five to thirty minutes.

Cook the bacon in a frying pan. Sauté the onions with the remaining coconut oil. Add the garlic, thyme, and mushrooms. Sauté until the mushrooms are tender, about five to ten minutes. Drain fat from pan, then add white wine, chicken broth, and cauliflower and bring to a boil. Reduce heat to a simmer for five minutes.

Blend soup with coconut oil in a food processor until you reach desired consistency. Return to low heat and add salt and pepper to taste.

Mushroom Coconut Soup

Ingredients:

  1 quart vegetable stock

  7 oz (200 g) chopped fresh mushrooms

  3 tablespoons virgin coconut oil

  1 medium onion, diced

  2 tablespoons thyme

  3 bay leaves

  5 large cloves garlic, minced

  ¼ cup white wine

  ⅓ cup plain flour

  1½ cups coconut milk

  1 teaspoon Himalayan salt (to taste)

  2 teaspoons fresh grind black pepper (to taste)

  2 tablespoons Thai fish sauce

Place chopped mushrooms in stock and simmer for twenty minutes.

Sauté the chopped onion in coconut oil in a heavy-bottom soup pot until the onions are transparent and golden.

Drain the stock from the mushrooms, reserving stock. Add the mushrooms to the sautéed onions. Add the thyme. Sauté for another five minutes or until tender. Add the bay leaves, minced garlic, and white wine, heating for another minute.

Place ½ cup reserved stock in a small saucepan and stir in flour over low heat until a paste forms. Add Thai fish sauce.

Add the rest of the stock and the coconut milk to the mushrooms in the soup pot. Heat until simmering, add the fish sauce paste, stirring until the soup thickens. Simmer for ten minutes, then remove bay leaves before serving.

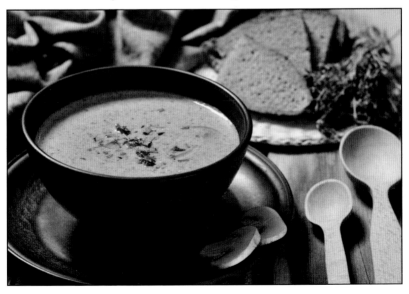

Thai Chicken Soup

Ingredients:

    2 green onions
    7 oz (200 g) mushrooms
    10 oz (300 g) baby corn, drained
    3½ oz (100 g) bamboo shoots, drained
    15 oz (500 g) chicken
    2 tablespoons coconut oil
    1 cup coconut butter plus 2 cups water
    2 cups chicken stock
    1 teaspoon curry powder
    ½ tablespoon honey
    2 teaspoon lemon juice
    Salt to taste

Finely chop vegetables and bamboo shoots. Dice chicken and fry in coconut oil in a large saucepan until cooked. Add onions and mushrooms and sauté for two minutes.

Add remaining ingredients and bring to a boil. Simmer for fifteen minutes.

Spicy Sweet Potato Soup

Ingredients:

    1 tablespoon coconut flour
    1 tablespoon virgin coconut oil
    1½ cups chicken stock
    1½ cups cubed sweet potato
    ¼ teaspoon fresh ginger

⅛ teaspoon ground cinnamon
⅛ teaspoon ground nutmeg
1 cup coconut milk
Salt and pepper to taste

Boil sweet potatoes until soft (about twenty minutes) and drain.

In a heavy saucepan, heat the virgin coconut oil, then stir in the coconut flour until the mixture combines into a caramel-colored roux. Add the chicken stock gradually, stirring until smooth after each addition. Bring to a boil, then lower to a simmer. Stir in the sweet potatoes and spices. Bring to a simmer again and cook for five minutes more.

In a blender, purée the soup in batches and return to the saucepan. Add the coconut milk and gently reheat the soup. Season with salt and pepper and serve.

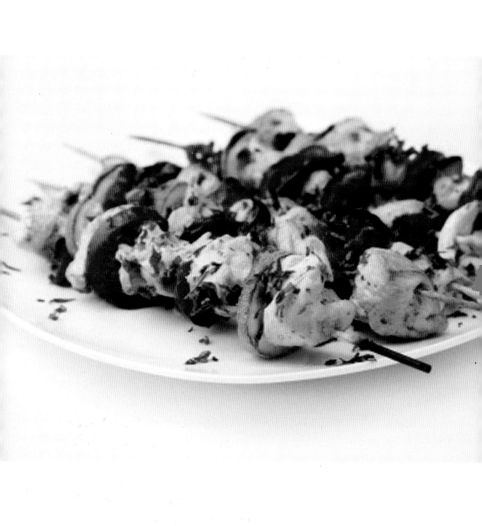

Dinner Recipes

Coconut Chicken Kebabs
Serves 3–6

Ingredients:

6 skewers

18 oz (500 g) raw chicken breast, cubed

1 cup freshly cut raw pineapple, cubed

⅓ cup coconut oil

½ cup shredded coconut

4 fresh, organic sweet peppers, chopped into a total of 24 pieces

2 tablespoons fresh lemon juice

Black pepper

1 cup large organic red onion slices

3 tomatoes cut into 8 pieces each

1 cup brown rice

Preheat oven to 355°F (180°C). When heated, place the chicken breast in the oven on a broiling pan. Cook for twenty-five to thirty minutes.

When the chicken is nearly cooked (fifteen minutes into cooking or so), heat a frying pan with a light film of coconut oil. Place the coconut oil, lightly cooked rice, and shredded coconut in the pan.

Attend to the frying pan carefully, when the chicken looks cooked (check the internal temperature to ensure it is above 160°F/70°C in the very center) begin slicing it into pieces about one-inch tall and wide, and about a half-inch thick. Add these to the skillet with the tomatoes and 2 tablespoons lemon juice. Let this simmer, stirring often for about twenty minutes.

Add the onion and sweet pepper; continue to add lemon juice and black pepper to taste.

Turn off the stove and oven.

Pierce a variety of the sliced pieces on each kebab, making sure it does not hold too much weight. Do not forget to include the fresh, cold pineapple.

Serve each kebab over a bowl of the cooked rice.

Coconut Lentil Stew

Ingredients:

    2 teaspoons expeller-pressed coconut oil
    ½ of a large yellow onion, chopped
    2 cups filtered water
    ½ teaspoon ginger, ground
    ½ teaspoon turmeric, ground
    1 cup yellow lentils, cooked
    1 tablespoons coconut palm sugar
    ½ tablespoon tamari
    ½ cup coconut, shredded

Heat coconut oil over medium heat in a large stockpot or saucepan. Sauté onion until browned, about six minutes. Add water, ginger, turmeric, lentils, coconut palm sugar, and tamari.

Bring to a boil then reduce to low heat. Simmer for about ten minutes to allow flavors to incorporate. Remove from heat and stir in shredded coconut.

Pan-Seared Halibut with Pineapple Salsa and Coconut Sauce

Ingredients

For the Salsa:
1 cup diced pineapple
½ small red onion, chopped
½ cup diced yellow, red, or orange bell pepper
Juice of ½ lime
Juice of ½ lemon
¼ bunch cilantro, chopped
Combine everything in a bowl and set aside.

For the Sauce:
½ cup extra virgin coconut oil
1 egg
½ cup chopped fresh cilantro
2 tablespoons chopped fresh parsley
Juice of ½ lime
Place everything in a blender and blend until smooth.

For the Fish:
Four 3-oz (85 g) halibut fillets
Himalayan sea salt and pepper, to taste
¼ cup coconut oil, divided
Garnish: 2 tablespoons of shaved coconut

Season the fish fillets with salt and pepper. Place 2 tablespoons coconut oil in a saucepan and heat over medium-high heat. Once hot, add the fish, cooking about four minutes on each side. Add up to 2 tablespoons more oil if needed, to prevent the fish from sticking to the pan. Remove from the pan, top with the salsa, drizzle with the sauce, garnish with the coconut shavings, and serve right away with a green salad.

Coconut Fried Chicken with Boiled Potatoes
Serves 4

Ingredients:
8 chicken pieces, thighs, breast, or drumstick, raw, organic, unfrozen
1 cup organic bread crumbs
½ cup dried, crispy onions
⅓ cup red wine vinegar
2 cups diced strawberries
1 cup fresh broccoli
4 medium-sized organic red potatoes, skinned
3 tablespoons lemon juice
⅗ cup coconut oil
¼ cup organic apricot preserves
½ cup olive oil
1 egg yolk
Mustard
Salt and pepper

Mix the red wine vinegar (leave a couple teaspoons behind for later use), diced strawberries, lemon juice, apricot preserves, and 1 tablespoon coconut oil. Mix these vigorously in an airtight container. Add the uncooked chicken pieces and allow to marinate overnight.

Heat the oven to 350°F (180°C). Mix the crispy onions and bread crumbs, and coat the marinated chicken in it.

Layer the remaining coconut oil at the bottom of a casserole dish. Add ¼ cup olive oil and stir.

Mix the crispy onions and bread crumbs, and coat the marinated chicken in it. Put the coated chicken in the dish and place it in the oven until it begins to fry. Steam broccoli until cooked.

For dipping sauce, mix the remaining coconut oil, red wine vinegar, and olive oil with the egg yolk.

For potatoes, bring a medium-sized pot of warm water to a boil and add peeled potatoes. Boil with salt, pepper, and lemon juice until soft.

Combine mustard, salt, and pepper to create a zesty mustard sauce, perfect for dipping.

Serve chicken with sauce, potatoes, and broccoli.

Slow-Cooked Coconut Beef Stroganoff

Ingredients:

  3 tablespoons coconut oil
  5 cloves garlic, minced
  1 large onion, chopped
  3 lbs (1.5 kg) sirloin tip roast, cut into strips
  Salt and pepper to taste
  1½ lbs (700 g) mushrooms, sliced
  1 tablespoon dill weed
  ½ cup red wine

½ cup beef or chicken stock
2 tablespoons coconut water vinegar
1 tablespoon Worcestershire sauce
3 tablespoons coconut flour
1 tablespoon tapioca flour/starch or cornstarch
2 cups sour cream
½ cup chopped fresh parsley

Grease the bottom of the slow cooker pot with extra coconut oil. Set aside.

Heat the 3 tablespoons of coconut oil in a frying pan and sauté garlic and onion lightly until browned and aromatic.

Place the beef strips in the slow cooker, and season with salt and pepper to taste. Place onion and garlic on top of beef, then add mushrooms and dill weed.

Mix together red wine, stock, coconut water vinegar, Worcestershire sauce, tapioca, and coconut flour in a small bowl, then pour over the beef. You can add more stock during cook time if desired.

Cover and cook on high for two hours. Stir in sour cream and parsley. Cook on low for 1½ hours until beef is tender.

Serve over pasta with extra sour cream and topped with extra parsley if desired.

Tropical Coconut Salmon

Ingredients:
¼ cup organic sugar
1½ tablespoons corn starch
2 lbs (1 kg) fresh salmon fillet

½ cup coconut oil
1 cup organic mango juice or pineapple juice
2 tablespoons organic fermented soy sauce
1–1½ cups coconut chips
Extra coconut oil for greasing pan
Preheat oven to 375°F (190°C).

Place salmon in a roasting pan greased with coconut oil and arrange coconut chips over salmon.

Mix together the organic sugar and cornstarch in a small bowl. In a small saucepan, melt ½ cup coconut oil over low heat. As it melts, add the mango juice and soy sauce. Stirring constantly, add the sugar mixture. Keep stirring until the mango sauce begins to thicken and then remove quickly from heat.

Pour the mango sauce on top of the salmon.

Bake for about fifteen minutes. To check if the salmon is done, gently pull at the fish a few inches from the edge. Once it is flaky and lighter in color, the salmon is done.

Coconut Citrus Tuna Steaks

Ingredients:

Extra virgin olive oil
Seafood seasoning blend of choice
1½ tablespoons coconut butter
1½ tablespoons lime juice
2 medium-sized tuna steaks
Virgin coconut oil

Rub both sides of the thawed tuna steaks with olive oil and seafood seasoning to coat. Mix equal parts softened coconut

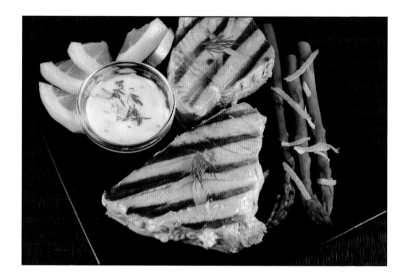

butter and fresh squeezed lime juice and beat with a fork until smooth and creamy.

Coat both sides of each steak with a thick layer of the coconut lime mixture. Allow to harden for a few seconds before flipping to coat the other side. Allow to marinate for ten minutes for flavors to absorb.

Preheat a frying pan coated with virgin coconut oil over medium heat for five minutes. Cook tuna steaks to desired doneness. Exact time will depend on the thickness of the individual steaks, but in general about two to three minutes per side produces a medium-rare tuna steak. I prefer to leave them fairly pink on the inside for maximum flavor and tenderness. Flip carefully to retain coating.

Serve immediately with rice and green vegetables.

Coconut Vegetable Ragout

Ingredients:

    4 teaspoons coconut oil
    1 bay leaf
    1 cinnamon stick
    2 cardamom pods
    3 green chilies, or adjust to your taste (slit vertically)
    ½ cup chopped onion
    1 cup mixed cut vegetables
    1 cup fresh coconut milk
    1½ cups water
    Salt, as needed
    1 teaspoon lemon juice
    Coriander for garnishing

Heat coconut oil in a pan. Add bay leaf, cinnamon, and cardamom. Sauté for two minutes and add chilies and onion. Fry until it turns golden brown.

Add the mixed vegetables and sauté for few minutes.

Dilute ½ cup of coconut milk with water and pour over the vegetables in the pan.

Add salt and cover the pan with a lid. Cook on medium heat until vegetables are softened. Remove from heat and add remaining coconut milk and lemon juice. Mix well and garnish with coriander. Serve with rice or Indian bread.

Carrots in Coconut Oil

Ingredients:

5–6 large fresh carrots
1 large yellow onion
Coconut oil
Butter
Salt, to taste

Wash and julienne the carrots. Slice onion into thin rings.

Heat the coconut oil and butter in a frying pan. Sauté the carrots and onions over high heat, until tender.

Add salt before serving, if desired.

Creamy Coconut Potato Mash

Ingredients:

2.2 lbs (1 kg) potatoes, unpeeled
¼ cup coconut oil
2 tablespoons butter or ghee
1 cup coconut milk, room temperature
Salt and pepper to taste

Steam the potatoes until very soft. Place them in a bowl, still with skins on, and add butter and oil. Mash the potatoes until smooth. Add the coconut milk and seasonings. Mash until well mixed.

Coconut Rice

Ingredients:

2 tablespoons virgin coconut oil
3 cups brown rice
1⅗ quarts water

1 fresh lime
½ cup dried unsweetened toasted coconut

Heat coconut oil and rice in pan. Stir constantly until rice darkens in color. Add water 2 cups at a time. Leave uncovered on high heat until it boils, then cover pan half way, and let cook for ten to fifteen minutes. Cover pan entirely, reduce temperature, and let simmer until rice is tender.

Fluff rice with fork and squeeze lime on top. Garnish with toasted coconut. Serve with chicken or fish.

Crispy Fish Fillets

Ingredients:

3 tablespoons coconut oil
¼ cup coconut flour
½ cup unsweetened shredded coconut
6 fresh or thawed white fish fillets
¼ cup coconut milk
Salt and pepper, to taste

Heat the coconut oil in a frying pan over medium-low heat.

Combine coconut flour and shredded coconut in a dish. Dip the fish in the coconut milk and then coat with coconut mixture. Sprinkle with salt and pepper and fry until golden brown.

Buttermilk Fish Fillets

Ingredients:

4 white fish fillets

1 cup buttermilk
⅓ cup coconut flour
¼ cup corn meal or seasoned fish fry mixture
⅓ cup panko (Japanese breadcrumbs)
Salt and pepper to taste
Dash cayenne pepper
1 cup coconut oil, divided
Juice from 2 or 3 lemons

Soak fillets in buttermilk. Mix all flours and spices together, and coat fillets in flour mixture.

Heat 2 tablespoons coconut oil on medium heat in a frying pan. Cook fillets until light brown on one side. While turning, add the other 2 tablespoons of coconut oil and brown on other side. Cook until fish is opaque and flakes easily.

Serve with fresh lemon juice squeezed over fish.

Spicy Coconut Fish

Ingredients:

2 tablespoons coconut oil
1 lb (500 g) fresh fish fillets
Cayenne pepper to taste
Salt
1 onion, diced
2 cloves garlic, minced
2 tablespoons coconut butter
1–2 cups water

Heat coconut oil in a frying pan. Season fish fillets and fry until lightly brown.

Remove fillets, and add onion, garlic, coconut butter, and 1–2 cups water to the pan. Bring to a boil for about ten minutes until mixture thickens slightly. Return fish fillets to the pan with coconut cream mixture. Cover pan and cook for an additional five minutes. Serve with rice and salad or steamed vegetables.

Spicy Fish Strips

Ingredients:

1 lb (500g) white fish
2 eggs, whisked
1 cup brown rice flour
¼ cup coconut flour
1 tablespoon achiote powder
1 tablespoon oregano
½ teaspoon cayenne powder
1 teaspoon freshly ground black pepper
1 teaspoon sea salt
½ cup coconut oil

Rinse fish fillets in cold water and then cut into short strips along lines of the fillets. Remove any bones.

Place eggs in one bowl. Mix together flours, spices, black pepper, and sea salt in another bowl.

Dip fish strips in eggs and then toss it in the flour mixture. Set them aside on a plate.

Warm up a ¼ cup of coconut oil in a large frying pan and heat oil on medium heat. Cook a few fish strips at a time, leaving plenty of room in the pan, until well browned on either side. Add fresh oil to pan between batches of fish. Set cooked fish aside on a plate lined with a paper towels.

Serve with freshly squeezed lime and tartar sauce.

Coconut Pilau

Ingredients:

- 3 cups coconut milk
- 1½ cups uncooked Basmati or long grain rice
- 1 tablespoon virgin coconut oil
- One 2-inch cinnamon stick, broken
- 3 clove buds
- 4 green cardamom crushed
- 1 star anise
- 1 bay leaf
- ½ teaspoon cumin seeds
- ½ teaspoon fennel seeds
- ¼ cup onions, thinly sliced
- 2 green chilies, slit
- 1 tablespoon ginger-garlic paste
- ½ teaspoon turmeric powder
- Salt to taste
- ¼ packed mint leaves, roughly chopped
- 1 tablespoon coconut flakes for garnish
- 1 tablespoon Golden raisins
- Fried shallots for garnish

Wash uncooked rice under running water and set aside.

Heat coconut oil in a large saucepan over medium-high heat. Add cinnamon, cloves, cardamoms, star anise, bay leaf, cumin seeds, and/or fennel seeds. Sauté for one minute until aromas are released.

Add sliced onions and slit green chilies and sauté until the onions are translucent. Add the ginger-garlic paste and sauté then season to taste with turmeric powder and salt.

Add uncooked basmati rice and mix gently to coat the rice grains with oil. Stir occasionally to keep the rice from sticking to the bottom of the pan.

Add the freshly prepared coconut milk into the pot with mint leaves and bring to a gentle boil. Stir once and cover the pot tightly with a lid. Simmer on medium heat for fifteen to twenty minutes until the liquid has been absorbed by the rice. When rice is done, each grain should be soft and should not clump.

Remove pot from heat, but keep covered until serving. Remove whole spices and garnish with roasted cashews and golden raisins. Serve with curry.

Ginger Pork Stir-fry

Ingredients:

1 lb (450 g) pork tenderloin, thinly sliced
2 red apples, thinly sliced
½ cup virgin coconut oil
1 tablespoon sesame oil
¼ cup honey
1 tablespoon shredded ginger
2 cups sliced mushroom
Salt and pepper to taste

1 chopped leek

2–3 cups of steamed wild rice

Sauté the oils with honey, pork, ginger, and apples for about eight minutes until the pork is cooked and apples are tender. Add the mushrooms and season with salt and pepper to taste. Sauté for another five minutes until the mushrooms are cooked. Serve on wild rice and garnish with the green onions.

Coconut Beef Curry

Serves 5

Preparation Time: 15 minutes

Ingredients:

1 small onion, diced

4 cloves garlic

Coconut oil, as needed for sautéing

1½ lbs (750 g) beef, sliced into strips

2 teaspoons curry

1 teaspoon cumin

1 teaspoon turmeric powder

Salt and pepper to taste

3 tablespoons coconut butter

2 cups beef broth

1 medium-sized sweet potato, cubed

1 medium-sized carrot, chopped

2 stalks celery, chopped

1 medium-sized zucchini, chopped

7 oz (200 g) mushrooms, sliced

Heat coconut oil and sauté onion and garlic until onion is soft. Add beef and sauté for another two minutes.

Add spices, coconut butter, and beef broth. Cover and simmer for two hours or until the meat is tender. Add remaining ingredients and continue cooking until the vegetables are soft and cooked through.

Serve over rice or pasta and top with sour cream or plain yogurt.

Crispy Fried Chicken

Ingredients:

2 cloves of garlic
1 onion, to taste
1 bunch shallots, finely chopped
6 raw macadamia nuts, crushed
1 teaspoon turmeric powder
3 teaspoons coriander powder
Coconut oil, as needed
Handful lime leaves
2 stalks lemon grass, bruised
¼ cup coconut milk
6 chicken drumsticks
1–2 cups shredded coconut flakes

Mix garlic, onions, shallots, macadamia nuts, turmeric, and coriander powder into a paste.

Heat coconut oil in a pan. Sauté the herb paste with lime leaves and lemon grass, until fragrant. Pour in the coconut milk and chicken drumsticks. Simmer for thirty minutes, or until sauce reduces into a paste. Remove from heat.

Preheat oven to 390°F (200°C). Roll the cooked drumsticks in the shredded coconut flakes until evenly coated. Place on a lined baking sheet and grill for about twenty minutes, turning once.

Serve with rice and salad.

Chicken Cacciatore

Ingredients:

- 1 whole chicken
- ½ cup virgin coconut oil
- 1 cup coconut flour
- 2½ cups sliced onions, thinly sliced
- ½ cup green pepper, chopped
- 2½ cloves garlic, crushed
- 15 oz (425 g) diced tomatoes
- 3½ tablespoons tomato paste
- 2 oz (50 g) sliced fresh mushrooms, drained
- 1¼ teaspoons Himalayan fine salt
- ⅓ teaspoon oregano

Wash chicken and pat dry. Separate into chicken pieces and coat in coconut flour. Heat virgin coconut oil in a frying pan and fry chicken over medium heat fifteen to twenty minutes until light brown. Remove chicken and set aside.

Add onion rings, green pepper, and garlic to the pan. Stir over medium heat until onion and pepper are tender. Stir in remaining ingredients.

Return chicken pieces to sauce. Place lid over the frying pan and simmer for thirty to forty minutes until chicken is tender.

Classic Coconut Chicken Curry

Ingredients:

- 1 whole chicken, cut into 6–8 pieces
- 3 tablespoons virgin coconut oil
- 2 tablespoons organic coconut flour
- $\frac{1}{2}$ teaspoon fine Himalayan salt
- $\frac{1}{4}$ teaspoon black pepper
- 1 tablespoon chopped fresh ginger root
- $\frac{1}{4}$ cup chopped onion
- 4 cloves garlic
- 1 tablespoon curry powder
- 2 cups chicken stock (you can use the neck and carcass to make this)
- $\frac{1}{4}$ cup water

Heat coconut oil in frying pan and sauté garlic, onion, and ginger. Add the chicken pieces, and brown slightly. Add chicken stock and simmer for fifteen minutes. Add spices and cover the pan. Continue cooking for another five minutes. Dissolve coconut flour in water and stir it into the pan. Cook for another five minutes.

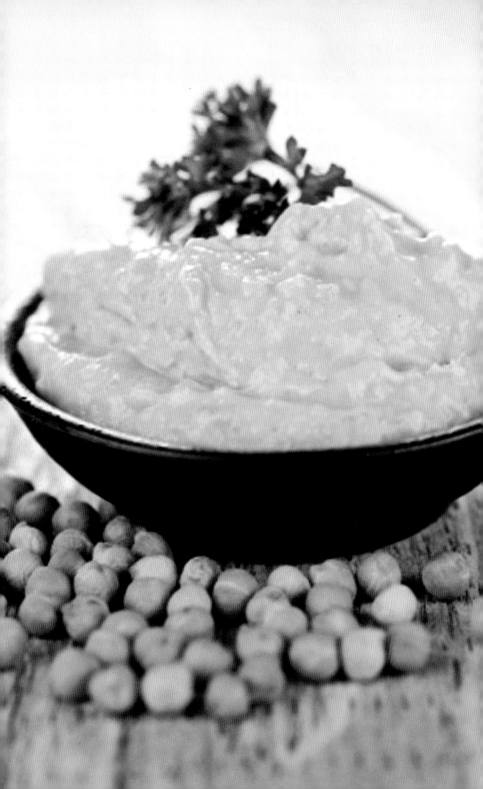

Condiments

Add a little more rejuvenating coconut oil to your daily diet with a splash of salad dressing or a side serving of sauce! You can even encourage your kids to increase their daily coconut oil intake by offering homemade chocolate hazelnut spread or ketchup! Coconut mayonnaise can be served as a spread or works as an excellent base for salad dressings. Combining olive oil with coconut oil for salad dressings will prevent the dressing from solidifying.

Hummus

Ingredients:

- ¼ cup softened coconut butter
- 2 garlic cloves, chopped
- 1½ cups garbanzo beans
- 2 tablespoons melted virgin coconut oil
- ½ scant teaspoon Himalayan salt
- ¼ cup water
- Lemon juice

In a blender, combine the softened coconut butter and garlic and add cooked, drained garbanzo beans. Pour in the melted coconut oil and sprinkle the Himalayan Salt over the center, then add the water.

Turn on the blender to pulse, stopping to push lumps into center, then repeating the pulsing action until smooth. Add lemon juice to taste.

Serve with vegetable crudités or corn chips.

Tomato Ketchup

Ingredients:

3 tablespoons coconut oil
1 white onion, roughly chopped
2–4 cloves garlic, peeled
¼ teaspoon celery seed
½ teaspoon allspice
½ teaspoon fennel seeds
3 whole cloves
Salt to taste
2 lbs (1 kg) tomatoes, quartered
¾ cup coconut water vinegar
2 tablespoons honey

Melt coconut oil in a large saucepan. Add onion and garlic and sauté lightly. Turn heat off and stir in remaining ingredients. Simmer over medium-low to low heat for approximately three hours, stirring regularly, until ketchup becomes thick and reduces by half.

Purée ketchup in a blender, then work it through a mesh strainer. Adjust seasoning to taste. If the ketchup isn't thick enough to taste, return to the saucepan and simmer until it reduces enough.

Cool and store in the refrigerator.

Italian Herb Dip

Ingredients:

½ cup coconut oil mayonnaise
½ cup Greek yogurt
½ cup coconut butter
¼ cup virgin palm oil
1 small clove garlic
1 tablespoon mixed Italian herbs

Process ingredients until creamy.

Coconut Mayonnaise

Ingredients:

1 whole egg
2 egg yolks
1 tablespoon mustard
1 tablespoon fresh lemon juice
½ teaspoon salt
¼ teaspoon pepper
½ cup melted virgin coconut oil
½ cup virgin olive oil

Blend eggs, mustard, lemon juice, salt, and pepper in a food processor for a few seconds.

Combine oils and place in a jug. With the processor running on low speed, add oils very slowly, first a few drops at a time, until combined. Then increase to a slow drizzle, then a thin steady stream. Continue until all oil is combined.

Coconut Barbeque Sauce

Ingredients:

½ cup coconut oil
½ cup apple cider vinegar
14 oz (400 g) Italian tomato pasta sauce
2 tablespoons chopped onion
1 teaspoon salt
¼ teaspoon dry mustard
¼ teaspoon celery seed
¼ teaspoon garlic powder
½ teaspoon sage
1 tablespoon raw honey

Combine all ingredients in saucepan. Bring to boil over medium-high heat, stirring occasionally. As soon as it boils, lower temperature and simmer for twenty to thirty minutes uncovered. Strain out onion bits if desired.

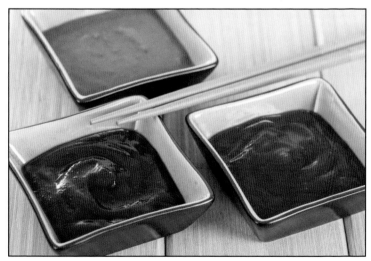

Dressings

Creamy Vinaigrette

Ingredients:

 ¼ cup red wine vinegar
 1 tablespoon finely chopped chives
 ½ teaspoon Himalayan Salt
 ½ tablespoon honey
 1 clove garlic, crushed
 Pinch oregano, basil and/or marjoram
 Pinch chili
 2 tablespoons coconut oil mayonnaise

In a small bowl, whisk together the vinegar, chives, salt, honey, garlic, and herbs. Add the mayonnaise and whisk until well blended. Refrigerate until ready to use.

Coconut and Olive Italian Dressing

Ingredients:

 ¼ cup coconut water vinegar
 2 tablespoons water
 ½ cup melted coconut oil
 ½ cup olive oil
 1 teaspoon salt
 Italian seasoning herbs to taste (oregano, marjoram, thyme, rosemary, basil, sage)

Whisk all ingredients together and serve over your favorite salad.

Honey Mustard Salad Dressing

Ingredients:
- ¼ cup homemade coconut mayonnaise
- ¼ cup mustard
- ½ cup raw honey
- ½ teaspoon coconut water vinegar

Blend all ingredients together in a small bowl. Serve over your favorite salad.

Garlic Vinaigrette
- 4–6 cloves of garlic
- ¼ cup melted coconut oil
- ¼ cup fermented organic soy sauce
- ¼ cup coconut water vinegar
- ¼ cup olive oil

Mince garlic until fine. Whisk together with the rest of the ingredients.

Store in a glass jar at room temperature. To strengthen the garlic flavor, allow the crushed garlic to sit in the dressing; alternately, strain the garlic out of the dressing. Shake well before serving.

Lemon Vinaigrette

Ingredients:

3 tablespoons fresh lemon juice
1 tablespoon honey
2 tablespoons finely minced red onion
½ teaspoon lemon zest
¼ teaspoon Himalayan salt
⅛ melted virgin coconut oil (melted if solid)
⅛ virgin olive oil

Blend oils and place in a jug. In a small bowl, whisk together all remaining dressing ingredients.

Holding jug high above the bowl, pour the oil in a thin, steady stream while whisking vigorously. Continue whisking until the mixture thickens.

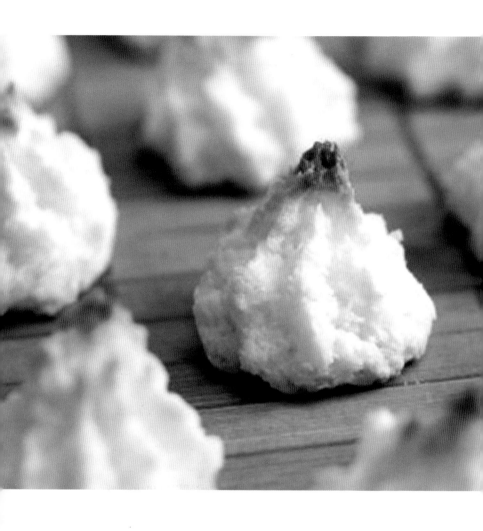

Desserts

Coconut Macaroons

Ingredients:
>   3 cups shredded coconut
>   1 teaspoon almond or vanilla extract
>   ⅛ teaspoon salt
>   ⅔ cup honey, melted slightly if solid
>   4 egg whites
>   1 teaspoon cream of tartar
>   Preheat oven to 355°F (180°C).

In a medium bowl, combine coconut, extract, and salt. Stir in honey until well combined.

Beat egg whites until stiff peaks form. Fold into coconut mixture along with cream of tartar.

Roll the mixture between your hands to make balls. Mixture should make twenty-two balls. Drop each ball onto the greased and lined baking tray and press it with your fingers. Bake for ten to fifteen minutes, or until browned.

Cool cookies on cookie sheet and dip into chocolate glaze.

Chocolate and Coconut Oil Pudding
Serves 4

Ingredients:

2 ripe avocados, sliced

½ cup raw cacao

7 dates (soaked in water for at least one hour, and water reserved)

½ cup raw honey

1½ teaspoons vanilla

3 tablespoons melted coconut oil

Pinch of Himalayan sea salt

Place everything in a blender or food processor and blend until smooth and fluffy. (You may need to add a little of the date-soaking water to create a creamy consistency.) Enjoy with fresh mango, peach, or apple slices for a great treat!

Coconut Pudding
Serves 2–4

Ingredients:

2 egg whites

⅓ cup rapadura

1½ cups coconut milk

1 tablespoon corn starch

1 teaspoon salt

¼ cup coconut oil

¼ cup coconut shavings

Place a shallow pot on the stovetop and add in egg whites. Turn the head about ¼ of the way up. Whisk the egg mixture, gradually adding the rapadura and coconut milk. Don't be generous with the milk, be sure to add it slowly so the whole batch doesn't turn into hot milk. Keep it as thick as possible.

Add corn starch and salt about a minute or two after the previous step. If the mixture starts to boil, turn the heat down. There should still be milk left at this point.

Wait between five and ten minutes before adding the coconut oil. We want the flavor to be introduced to the dish as late as possible. Continue adding the milk slowly. There should be roughly a half cup left, depending on how accepting the mixture is.

Add the coconut oil 1 tablespoons at a time in addition to the remainder of the coconut milk. If all else fails, add a touch of regular milk.

When the ingredients are completely mixed and there are no visible traces of raw eggs, turn the stove down a notch. Wait two minutes just to be sure.

Let the mixture cool and place it in the refrigerator for up to an hour. When the mixture is cold, add coconut shavings if desired.

Coconut Tapioca Rice
Serves 6

Ingredients:

2 tablespoons butter or butter substitute
¼ cup tapioca pearls
½ cup rice
1 cup coconut milk

1 cup almond milk (any flavor)
½ cup rapadura
¼ cup coconut oil
¼ cup raisins
¼ cup coconut shavings
½ cup diced apples
½ cup long grain rice

Place the coconut milk in a large pot and put the stove on low heat. As soon as the milk begins to foam, add the tapioca pearls. It is incumbent that these cook while the rice portion is prepared. Be sure to stir this constantly.

Put the pan on medium-low heat, only slightly higher than the pot. Add the butter, followed by the rice. Slowly add the milk as the butter-rice mixture adapts. At this point, add 1–2 tablespoons coconut oil in addition to the rapadura. This will take at least five minutes to cook. Move the ingredients around in the pan as much as possible. After five minutes, add 1 tablespoon coconut oil to the pan and the remaining oil to the large pot. Stir thoroughly.

The pan mixture will be visibly finished when the rice begins to lose its shape. This is a tricky step, as you do not want it to lose its texture completely. Try to turn off the burner as soon as it appears to be softening. At this point, check the status of the tapioca coconut mixture.

The pearls in the tapioca mixture should be soft and tender. The total cooking time for the pot should be roughly twenty minutes.

This is the most complex step and is therefore the most vulnerable to mistakes. Any excess milk from either pan/pot

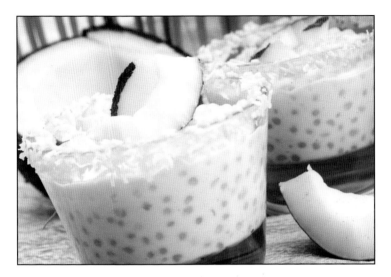

should be drained before attempting this. Add the rice mixture into the pot. Do not add heat. It is important that the mixtures are cooked to similar textures, otherwise one will immediately invade the other.

Assuming the transfer went well, the coconut tapioca and rice pudding should be mixed in a large pan with a minimal amount of liquid. Place this back on the stove on extremely low heat. Stir slowly for about fifteen minutes, carefully allowing the mixtures to take a liking to each other. If all goes well, it is time to add toppings and celebrate.

Leaving the heat as low as possible, add the raisins, followed by the shredded coconut, and finally the diced apples. Mix these toppings completely and serve the dish warm. While cold tapioca can be tasty, the cold rice pudding will not complement it at all.

Coconut Oil and Cocoa Fudge

Ingredients:
- ½ cup of virgin coconut oil
- ½ cup of coconut sugar paste
- ½ cup of organic cocoa powder
- Pinch sea salt
- ½ teaspoon vanilla extract

In a heat-resistant glass measuring cup, add the coconut oil. Fill a small saucepan with a few inches of water and place the glass measuring cup in it. Heat on the stove top until the coconut oil is mostly melted (the coconut oil should be room temperature, not hot).

In a food processor using the regular blade, add the melted coconut oil and the rest of the ingredients and mix until well combined.

Place parchment paper in a loaf pan to cover the bottom and sides of the pan. Scrape your fudge mix into the loaf pan and fold the parchment paper over the top of the fudge. Gently press down to even out the thickness of the fudge (you want it to be about half an inch thick, and it will cover probably about half of the bottom of your loaf pan). Take out the fudge and place in the freezer or refrigerator until it has set. In the freezer it only takes about twenty to thirty minutes.

Cut into small squares—enjoy!

Chocolate Apricot Bites

Ingredients:

⅓ cup brown rice syrup
2 tablespoons coconut oil, melted
1 tablespoon almond butter
1 teaspoon vanilla extract
1½ cups oats
1 tablespoon cocoa powder
¼ cup almonds, chopped
¼ cup dried apricots, chopped
¼ cup chocolate chips

Preheat oven to 330°F (165°C).
Combine the brown rice syrup, oil, almond butter, and vanilla in a large bowl until well-mixed. Fold in the oats and add the rest of the ingredients, stirring to coat.

Once the mixture is well combined, pour onto a lined baking sheet and bake for twenty-two minutes in a preheated oven, stirring once.

Chocolate Avocado Pudding

Ingredients:

2 ripe avocados
½ cup raw honey
½ cup organic cocoa powder
2 tablespoons coconut oil, melted
1 teaspoon organic vanilla extract

Purée the mashed avocados in a blender. Add remaining ingredients and blend until smooth and glossy.

Chocolate Maple Brownies

Ingredients:

1 cup coconut butter
2–3 eggs
½ cup honey
½ teaspoon baking soda
¼ teaspoon Himalayan salt
1½ teaspoons organic vanilla extract
¼ cup cocoa powder
⅓ cup chocolate chips
¼ cup chopped walnuts

Preheat oven to 355°F (180°C). Grease a 9 x 9 or 12 x 8-inch pan.

In a large bowl, measure out all ingredients and mix until combined. Pour into a prepared pan and bake twenty to twenty-five minutes until the top is slightly crisp and the middle is soft.

Icy Almond Fudge

Ingredients:

2 cups raw creamy almond butter (unsalted)
½ cup coconut oil, softened
3 tablespoons raw honey
1 teaspoon fine sea salt

Bring all ingredients to room temperature for an hour before preparation. Mix all the ingredients together in a medium bowl, until smooth and creamy.

Transfer the mixture to a square baking dish lined with baking paper, and smooth the top with a spatula. Freeze until solid (about an hour). Remove the fudge by lifting the paper out of the pan, then cut into squares and serve immediately.

Store in the freezer to maintain texture.

Coconut Rice Cakes

Ingredients:

   1½ cups cooked long grain rice
   ¼ cup warm water
   ½ teaspoon baking powder
   ½ teaspoon salt
   1 teaspoon freshly grated nutmeg
   1 teaspoon honey
   1 cup organic unbleached all-purpose flour
   ¼ cup coconut flour
   3 eggs, beaten
   2 tablespoons coconut oil
   1 tablespoon powdered sugar

Place the rice and warm water in a mixing bowl and mash the rice. Add the baking powder, salt, nutmeg, and honey and mix well. Mix the two flours together, then, alternate adding the flour and eggs to the rice mixture. Mix until smooth.

Heat the coconut oil in a large frying pan. Drop the rice mixture by level tablespoons into the hot oil. Cook four minutes on each side or until golden brown.

Transfer to paper towels and let them dry. Sprinkle with powdered sugar.

Coconut Carrot Cake

Ingredients:

3 cups shredded carrots
1½ cups whole wheat flour, fresh ground if possible
½ cup coconut flour
¼ cup whole organic sugar
3 teaspoons baking soda
1½ teaspoons baking powder
½ teaspoon salt
1 teaspoon cinnamon
¾ cup pecans (optional)
¾ cup dried shredded coconut (optional)
4 eggs
1½ cups honey
1½ cups warm liquid coconut oil
1¼ teaspoons vanilla
225 g crushed pineapple with juice

Preheat oven to 355°F (180°C).
Combine all dry ingredients together in a large bowl. Add all remaining ingredients and stir until well-combined. Pour into an un-greased 9 x 13-inch (23 x 33 cm) baking pan and bake for fifty minutes or until tester inserted in the center of cake comes out clean. Cool.

To make Coconut Cream Icing, beat together ½ cup coconut butter, ½ cup butter, and ¾ cup honey. Drizzle over cake.

Chocolate Glaze

Ingredients:

¾ cup chopped chocolate or chips, about 4.5 oz
1½ tablespoons coconut oil
1½ tablespoons butter
1 tablespoon brown rice syrup
¼ teaspoon vanilla extract

Combine chocolate, coconut oil, butter, and syrup in a double boiler and melt gently. Once mixture is smooth, add vanilla.

Coconut Pie

Ingredients:

Dairy-Free Whole Wheat Crust:
1 cup whole wheat flour
½ cup unbleached all-purpose flour
2 teaspoon sugar
½ teaspoon sea salt
½ cup coconut oil
¼ cup plus 2 tablespoons coconut milk

Coconut Pie Filling:
1 cup organic sugar
2 eggs
¼ cup coconut flour
¼ cup plus 1 tablespoon coconut oil
½ cup coconut milk
1½ cups shredded unsweetened dried coconut
1 teaspoon vanilla extract

Crust:

Mix dry ingredients together. Add coconut oil. Use a pastry cutter to cut the oil into the dry ingredients. Add coconut milk a little at a time until the dough is firm and pliable. Turn on a floured surface and knead several times. Roll dough into a circle with an 8.5-inch (22 cm) circumference. Transfer to a pie plate and press into place, using fingers if necessary.

Pie Filling:

Preheat oven to 355°F (180°C).

Mix together sugar and eggs. Add oil and flour and mix well. Add coconut milk and fold in 1 cup coconut. Add vanilla and mix well. Sprinkle remaining coconut on top of the pie. Pour into your whole wheat pie crust.

Bake in preheated oven for fifty to fifty-five minutes.

Lemon Rosemary Cake

Ingredients:

2 large eggs, separated
¼ cup honey
¼ cup coconut oil, plus extra for greasing the pan
1 tablespoon fresh lemon zest
1 tablespoon finely chopped rosemary
1 cup blanched almond flour
¼ cup arrowroot starch
½ teaspoon baking soda
¼ teaspoon sea salt
Sliced almonds, for sprinkling

Preheat oven to 355°F (180°C). Lightly grease 18 cups of a mini muffin tin with coconut oil.

Beat egg whites to soft peaks. Set aside.

In a small saucepan, melt honey and oil together until just melted.

Transfer to a small bowl and whisk in lemon zest, rosemary, and egg yolks.

In a medium bowl, whisk together almond flour, arrowroot, baking soda, and sea salt. Stir in the oil and honey mixture to form a thick batter.

Fold the egg whites into the batter using a metal spoon until thoroughly combined and batter is a pale golden color.

Spoon batter evenly among the greased muffin cups. Sprinkle tops with almonds.

Bake for ten to twelve minutes until the cakes are golden brown and a toothpick inserted comes out clean. Cool completely before removing from pan and serving.

Non-dairy Coconut Cream

Ingredients:

½ cup raw cashews, soaked
3 tablespoons honey
2 tablespoons coconut butter
½ vanilla bean (or 1½ teaspoons vanilla extract)
½ teaspoon lemon juice
Pinch salt
½ cup filtered water
Additional water, as needed to thin

Combine all ingredients in a high-speed blender and blend until smooth. (If you don't have coconut butter, leave it out and stream in 1 tablespoon of melted coconut oil at this point, with the blender running.) Add more water, a tablespoon at a time, as needed to blend to a drizzly consistency. Serve over fresh berries or chopped fruit.

Honey Chocolate Fudge Spread

Ingredients:

    3 tablespoons unsalted butter
    3 tablespoons raw honey (or to taste)
    3 tablespoons virgin coconut oil
    2 tablespoons cocoa powder
    $\frac{1}{4}$ teaspoon cinnamon
    2 teaspoons vanilla extract
    $\frac{1}{4}$ teaspoon salt (or to taste)

Cut butter into chunks and place in a medium saucepan along with honey and coconut oil. Melt over low heat and whisk to combine. Add the remaining ingredients and whisk the mixture thoroughly to combine.

Taste and adjust honey and/or salt if necessary. Extra salt will enhance the chocolate flavor if required. Cool the sauce then store in fridge in a glass jar. As the fudge sets, it will become the consistency of peanut butter and can be used as a spread for bread, pancakes, or waffles. Alternately, heat until it takes the consistency of sauce and pour over ice cream.

Coconut Strawberry Tart

Ingredients:

Crust:

1 cup raw macadamia nuts, pecans, or walnuts
¼ cup dates, pitted
⅓ cup dried coconut

For the custard:

2 cups chopped cashews or pine nuts soaked for at least half an hour
½ cup lemon juice (or lime juice)
½ cup honey
½ cup coconut oil
1 teaspoon vanilla
¼ teaspoon sea salt

For the topping:

Sliced strawberries or fruit of choice.

Crust: Process the nuts and dates in the food processor. Sprinkle coconut on the bottom of a tart pan and press crust onto the coconut.

Custard: Heat coconut oil gently until softened. Mix coconut oil with cashews, lemon, honey, vanilla, and salt until well combined and smooth.

Pour the mixture onto the crust. Tap the bottom of the pan gently to remove any air bubbles.

Freeze until almost firm. Top with sliced strawberries, or fruit of choice. Return to the freezer for another fifteen minutes until firm. Serve immediately.

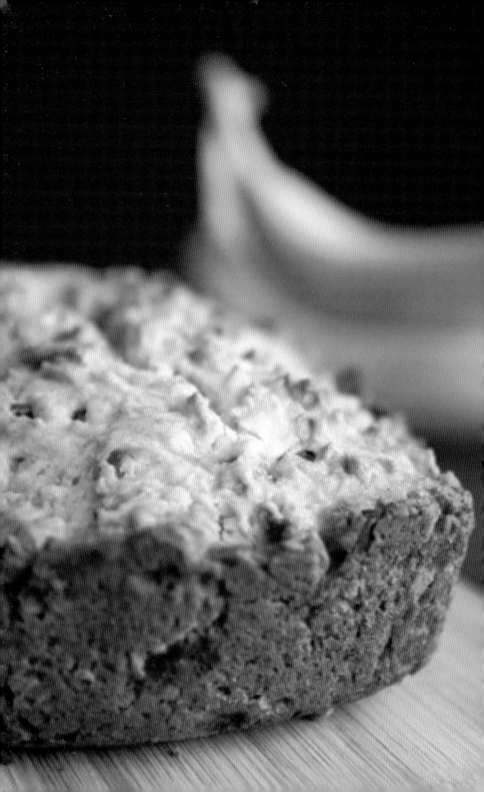

Breads, Cookies, and Muffins

Enhance the health benefits of your favorite home-baked treat by replacing butter with coconut oil. For extra coconut goodness, incorporate coconut flour and coconut flakes. If you want to replace butter with coconut oil in your own favorite recipe, you need exactly the same amount.

Super Moist Banana Bread

Ingredients:

1½ cups plain/all-purpose flour
1 teaspoon baking soda
1 teaspoon baking powder
Pinch salt
½ cup virgin coconut oil
1 cup cream cheese
1 cup brown sugar
1 egg
2 medium-sized bananas

Heat oven to 350°F (175°C). Line a loaf pan with baking paper.

Sift the dry ingredients together in a large mixing bowl and set aside. In a separate bowl, beat the coconut oil on medium speed until soft. Add the cream cheese and continue beating for three minutes. Add the sugar and continue beating for five minutes or until the mixture is light and fluffy. Mix in the bananas and egg until well combined. Add the dry ingredients and mix with a wooden spoon until combined. Pour the mixture into the loaf pan.

Bake for forty-five to fifty-five minutes until the loaf is golden brown. To test whether the loaf is cooked, press your finger into the center. If the indentation springs back, the loaf is cooked.

Apple Walnut Bread

Ingredients:

    $1\frac{3}{4}$ cups pastry flour
    1 teaspoon baking powder
    $\frac{1}{2}$ teaspoon baking soda
    $\frac{1}{2}$ teaspoon salt
    $\frac{1}{2}$ cup virgin coconut oil
    1 cup whole sugar
    2 eggs
    $\frac{1}{4}$ cup brandy
    1 cup shredded apples
    $\frac{1}{2}$ cup coconut flakes
    $\frac{1}{2}$ cup chopped raisins
    $\frac{1}{2}$ cup chopped walnuts, more to taste

Preheat oven to 355°F (180°C). Grease and flour a 5 x 9-inch (13 x 23 cm) bread pan.

Sift the first four ingredients together and set aside. Cream the oil and sugar until light and fluffy. Add eggs one at a time, beating well after each addition. Stir brandy and apples into the wet mixture, then stir in sifted flour until just combined. Gently fold coconut, raisins, and walnuts into mixture. Do not over-mix.

Spread mixture evenly in the pan and bake for one hour. To test whether the bread is ready, gently press the center of the loaf—it should spring back. Allow to cool for ten minutes in the pan, then use a butter knife to gently loosen the edges and turn it out on a cooling rack to cool completely. Cuts best with a serrated knife and gentle sawing motion when cool.

Zucchini Bread

Ingredients:

3 eggs
1 cup virgin coconut oil
1 cup raw honey
1 teaspoon vanilla extract
2 cups grated zucchini
3 cup whole wheat flour
3 teaspoons cinnamon
1 teaspoon salt
¼ teaspoon baking powder
1 teaspoon baking soda

Preheat oven to 355°F (180°C). Grease two loaf pans with extra coconut oil and set aside.

Sift flour with cinnamon, baking powder, and baking soda. Make a well in the center.

Beat eggs, oil, honey, and vanilla extract together until well blended and pour into well in the flour. Mix until just combined. Stir grated zucchini through batter.

Pour into prepared pans and bake for fifty to sixty minutes.

Coconut Chocolate Chip Cookies

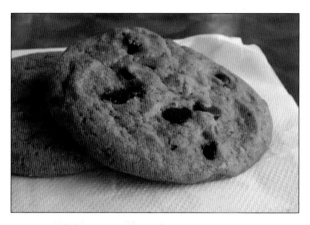

Ingredients:

 2 tablespoons coconut flour
 ¼ teaspoon unrefined sea salt
 3–4 tablespoons sugar
 ¼ teaspoon baking soda
 2 tablespoons unsweetened coconut flakes
 ⅓ cup coconut oil, melted and cooled
 2 large eggs
 ¼ cup chocolate chips

Preheat oven to 350°F (175°C). Place a sheet of baking paper on a baking tray.

Combine coconut flour, salt, sugar, baking soda, and coconut flakes in a large bowl and stir well. Make a well in the center.

Combine eggs and coconut oil, then pour into well in dry ingredients. Mix together until smooth. Set aside for five minutes before folding in chocolate chips.

Drop heaped tablespoonfuls onto the baking tray. Bake for twelve to fourteen minutes.

Raspberry Banana Cookies

Makes about three dozen bite-sized cookies

Ingredients:

3 large, ripe bananas, well mashed (about 1½ cups)

½ cup raspberries

1 teaspoon vanilla extract

¼ cup coconut oil, melted 2 cups rolled oats

⅔ cup almond meal

⅓ cup coconut, finely shredded and unsweetened

½ teaspoon cinnamon

½ teaspoon fine grain sea salt

1 teaspoon baking powder

6–7 oz (150 g) chocolate chips or dark chocolate bar chopped

Preheat oven to 350°F (175°C). Line a baking tray with baking paper.

Combine the bananas, vanilla extract, and coconut oil. Set aside. In a separate bowl whisk together the oats, almond meal, shredded coconut, cinnamon, salt, and baking powder. Add the oats mixture to the banana mixture and stir until combined.

Fold the raspberries and chopped chocolate into the mixture. Drop half a tablespoon of dough onto the baking tray, placing each dollop about five centimeters apart.

Bake for twelve to fourteen minutes.

Buttermilk Cookies

Ingredients:

1 cup whole wheat flour
1 cup unbleached plain flour
1 tablespoon baking powder
¼ teaspoon baking soda
¾ teaspoon salt
⅓ cup virgin coconut oil, solid
¾ cup buttermilk

Preheat the oven to 440°F (230°C) and cover a baking tray with baking paper. Sift together flours, baking powder and soda, and salt. Roughly cut coconut oil into small chunks and toss it through the flour. Gently stir buttermilk into flour mixture until just combined into a dough. (Do *not* over mix or cookies will be tough).

Gently roll dough until it is ¾ of an inch (2 cm) thick. Only roll once or the dough will toughen. Cut into cookies with a sharp cookie cutter and place on a baking tray. Bake for about ten minutes until the cookies are golden brown on the outside and tender on the inside. Cool before eating.

Coconut Gingerbread Men

Ingredients:

½ teaspoon salt
½ teaspoon baking soda
1½ teaspoons ground ginger

1 teaspoon cinnamon
½ teaspoon cloves
½ teaspoon nutmeg
3 cups whole wheat flour
⅔ cup black strap molasses
⅓ cup coconut oil

Preheat oven to 355°F (180°C). Place baking paper over baking tray.

Mix all dry ingredients together and make a well in the center. Slowly add oil to molasses and blend slowly. Pour into well in the center of the dry ingredients and stir to combine. The mixture should make firm, pliable dough.

Roll dough out, splashing with water if it seems too dry. Cut into gingerbread men, using a cookie cutter.

Bake for eight to ten minutes. Ice to decorate.

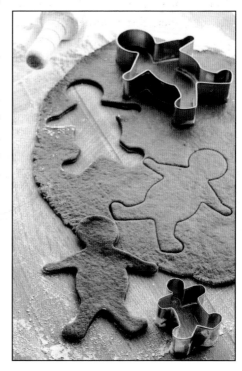

Cherry Coconut Cookies

Makes 24 large cookies

Ingredients:

6 eggs
½ cup coconut oil
1 teaspoon vanilla
⅔ cup maple syrup
1 teaspoon baking soda
1 cup quick rolled oats
1 cup coconut flakes
⅓ cup coconut flour
1 cup glace cherries or dried unsweetened cranberries

Preheat oven to 355°F (180°C). Place a sheet of baking paper over a baking tray.

Blend eggs, oil, vanilla, and maple syrup. Add baking soda. Add quick oats, coconut flakes, and cranberries. Fold in flour until just combined.

Drop tablespoons of dough onto baking tray.

Bake for fourteen minutes or until edges start to brown. Cool on wire rack.

Coconut Cookies

Serves 4–8

Ingredients:

1 cup organic white spelt flour
¼ cup butter
4 tablespoons coconut oil
½ cup rapadura

1 egg yolk (or egg substitute)
1 full egg (or egg substitute)
1 teaspoon baking powder
⅓ cup shredded coconut
2 teaspoons pineapple juice

Preheat oven to 325°F (160°C). Mix all the dry ingredients. Whisk the butter, slowly adding the coconut oil and egg/egg yolk.

Add the dry mixture to the mixing batch, and begin creating small dough balls, no more than an inch in diameter. Once the oven is thoroughly heated, place the dough balls in the oven on a pan with a baking sheet. Be sure they are spaced at least an inch apart.

They should be ready in fifteen minutes and ready to eat just a couple minutes after that.

Almond Berry Muffins

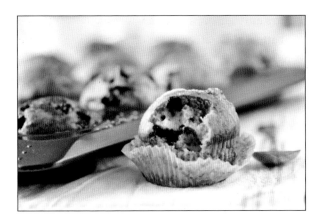

Ingredients:

3 eggs
2 tablespoons melted coconut oil
3 tablespoons maple syrup
2 tablespoons coconut milk
¼ teaspoon salt
½ teaspoon vanilla extract
½ teaspoon almond extract
½ cup coconut flakes
¼ cup packed coconut flour
½ cup packed almond flour
¼ teaspoon baking soda
1 cup blackberries, blueberries, or raspberries

Blend coconut flakes in food processor until fine. Set aside.

Blend eggs, oil, coconut milk, maple syrup, salt, vanilla, and almond extract.

Sift flours and baking soda, and stir in coconut flakes. Fold flours into batter and gently stir in the berries. Spoon batter into muffin cups.

Bake at 400°F (205°C) for twenty minutes for regular-sized muffins.

Raspberry Oat Muffins

Ingredients:

1½ cups rolled oats
2 teaspoons baking powder
½ teaspoon sea salt
1 teaspoon cinnamon
2 tablespoons maple syrup
1 egg
⅓ cup coconut oil, melted
½ teaspoon vanilla extract
½ teaspoon almond extract
½ cup buttermilk
½ cup shredded coconut
2 cups raspberries (fresh or frozen)

Preheat oven to 400°F (205°C). Grease muffin tins with nonstick cooking spray or place paper cups in tin and set aside.

In a large bowl, combine rolled oats, baking powder, salt, and cinnamon. Make a well in the center.

In another bowl, whisk egg, syrup, coconut oil, and buttermilk and pour the mix into the well in the dry ingredients. Add vanilla and almond flavoring and stir until combined. Fold in raspberries and shredded coconut.

Spoon into muffin cups and bake for twenty minutes until golden brown.

Index